C000273089

Fatal Protein

Fatal Protein

The Story of CJD, BSE, and Other Prion Diseases

Rosalind M. Ridley
and
Harry F. Baker
Department of Experimental Psychology,
University of Cambridge

Oxford New York Tokyo
OXFORD UNIVERSITY PRESS
1998

Oxford University Press, Great Clarendon Street, Oxford OX2 6DP

Oxford New York

Athens Auckland Bangkok Bogota Bombay
Buenos Aires Calcutta Cape Town Dar es Salaam
Delhi Florence Hong Kong Istanbul Karachi
Kuala Lumpur Madras Madrid Melbourne
Mexico City Nairobi Paris Singapore
Taipei Tokyo Toronto Warsaw

and associated companies in
Berlin Ibadan

Oxford is a trade mark of Oxford University Press

Published in the United States
by Oxford University Press, Inc., New York

© Rosalind M. Ridley and Harry F. Baker, 1998

All rights reserved. No part of this publication may be
reproduced, stored in a retrieval system, or transmitted, in any
form or by any means, without the prior permission in writing of Oxford
University Press. Within the UK, exceptions are allowed in respect of any
fair dealing for the purpose of research or private study, or criticism or
review, as permitted under the Copyright, Designs and Patents Act, 1988, or
in the case of reprographic reproduction in accordance with the terms of
licences issued by the Copyright Licensing Agency. Enquiries concerning
reproduction outside those terms and in other countries should be sent to
the Rights Department, Oxford University Press, at the address above.

This book is sold subject to the condition that it shall not,
by way of trade or otherwise, be lent, re-sold, hired out, or otherwise
circulated without the publisher's prior consent in any form of binding
or cover other than that in which it is published and without a similar
condition including this condition being imposed
on the subsequent purchaser.

A catalogue record for this book is available from the British Library

Library of Congress Cataloging in Publication Data
(Data available)

ISBN 0 19 852435 8

Typeset by Joshua Associates Ltd., Oxford
Printed in Great Britain by
St. Edmundsbury Press, Suffolk

'Human history becomes more and more a race between education and catastrophe.'

The outline of history; being a plain history of life and mankind
(H. G. Wells 1920)

Preface

Sometime in the middle of the 1980s, before bovine spongiform encephalopathy (BSE) had made its entrance on to the stage, we were asked for advice by a family general practitioner. He had been consulted by one of his patients who, although in good health, was concerned about her future. She told him that her mother and her grandmother had both died in early middle age, and that in each case the diagnosis had been Creutzfeldt–Jakob disease (CJD). She wanted to know whether she was likely to get the same disease. The doctor vaguely remembered something from his student days about unusual viruses and cannibalism, although he felt certain that the latter was unlikely to be a consideration in his patient's case. He approached us because he had recently seen an article published by us and our colleague, Tim Crow, in the *British Medical Journal*, about the demonstration of a transmissible agent in a genetically inherited variant of Creutzfeldt–Jakob disease. We had been working with a large family in south-east England in which this variant, Gerstmann–Sträussler–Scheinker disease (GSS), is inherited in the same way as the rather better known Huntington's disease. In this pattern of inheritance, the disease has a 50 per cent chance of appearing in the offspring if one of the parents is affected. Since the worried patient hailed from the same part of Britain, we were not surprised to discover that she also belonged to this large family.

At that time the spongiform encephalopathies, or, as they later became known, the prion diseases, were almost completely unknown to the general public. The human prion diseases were, and still are, extremely rare. Each year in Britain about 500 000 people die, mostly of heart attacks, strokes, or cancer, and, at present, as many as 150 000 elderly people are suffering from Alzheimer's disease. These large numbers can be contrasted with the approximately 50 people in Britain who succumb to prion disease each year, a rate of one case per million of the population. This very low rate is approximately constant throughout the world: yet by 1996 everyone had heard of CJD. So what had happened? The answer, of course, is BSE.

When the first cases of this new neurological disease in cattle appeared, the veterinarians recognized that the brain pathology was similar to that seen in scrapie, a fatal neurological disease of sheep, known in Europe since the middle of the eighteenth century, and endemic in British flocks. A relatively small number of scientists around the world were trying to understand the biology of the prion diseases because they seemed unlike any other disease and held the promise of revolutionizing the way in which some basic mechanisms of infection were considered. But more of that later. With the advent of BSE, we spent a lot of time lecturing to groups of veterinarians about the human prion diseases and, in so doing, learnt something about animal diseases and farming practices. What we found puzzling, however, was the lack of reconciliation between research findings in the areas of human and animal prion diseases despite the seminal letter to the journal, *Lancet*, in 1959, by the veterinarian Bill Hadlow, which drew attention to the similarities between these diseases. His suggestion that the human prion disease, kuru, like scrapie, might be experimentally transmissible, led eventually to Carleton Gajdusek being awarded the Nobel prize in 1976. Gajdusek and his colleagues showed that if brain tissue from a patient who had died from kuru, or from CJD, was injected directly into the brain of a chimpanzee, the animal would itself develop spongiform encephalopathy some time later. In *Laughing death*, the autobiographical account of his participation in the discovery of kuru in the 1950s, Vincent Zigas remarks that there was some surprise amongst academics that the Nobel prize was not awarded jointly to Gajdusek and Hadlow.

Despite this clear intersection between research on scrapie and kuru, it was the case, even in the early 1980s, that veterinarians ignored research findings from the human field, and clinicians were often unaware of developments in the animal world. This failure to engage led to contradictions which even today have not been fully resolved. One such is the matter of maternal transmission of disease, which, most clinicians accept, does not happen in human prion disease. However, despite the detailed arguments by veterinary scientist James Parry to the contrary, it has been widely accepted by the veterinary profession that maternal transmission of scrapie is an important factor in maintaining scrapie as an endemic disease.

The great controversy besetting the world of the spongiform encephalopathies remains the nature of the transmissible agent. Those who support the protein-only hypothesis have yet to explain how a protein can transmit disease from one animal to another, while those who maintain that a transmissible agent must contain its own nucleic acid have yet to provide evidence for the existence of such a nucleic acid. Even those scientists not directly involved in research in this area find themselves supporting one side or the other, since these conflicting viewpoints appeal to the conservative or adventurous side in all of us. But this does result in conflict. One of the most distinguished and controversial players in recent years, Stanley Prusiner, included a quotation in the volume *Prion diseases of humans and animals*, which he edited with colleagues in 1992: 'At every crossway on the road that leads to the future, tradition has placed against each of us ten thousand men to guard the past' (Maurice Maeterlinck, 1862–1949).

Although the emergence of BSE and the deaths of more than 160 000 cattle between 1986 and 1996 has thrust these strange diseases into the limelight, there has been quiet progress in our understanding of the science since the early 1980s. Quiet, that is, as far as the public is concerned, but far from quiet for the scientists involved. It is astonishing that such a relatively small field has produced such a vociferous and argumentative group of researchers! The characters involved are often larger than life, physically as well as intellectually, and the research arena ranges from the highlands of Papua New Guinea to the lowlands of Scotland. Yet, despite the many different schools of opinion in the prion diseases, the scientists have, with a few notable exceptions, been able to enjoy the cut and thrust of the arguments. When we first came into the field in late 1979, the small numbers actively researching in the area formed what scrapie researcher, Richard Kimberlin, called the 'club'. Things are very different now. The field has grown enormously in the past 10 years. Prion disease research has become big business, with research groups sprouting up in all parts of the world. With the emergence of the new variant form of CJD and the possibility that it may be due to eating BSE-infected meat, prion disease has become an important issue of public health and there are very real fears that we may see a major epidemic of human disease. This has stimulated prion disease research still further.

In this short account of prion diseases we hope to be able to give the reader some idea of the exciting science that has been, and is being, done, and why it is so important. The reader might also begin to understand why it is that those who work in the prion diseases become so obsessed. We hope that this book will appeal to scientists and non-scientists alike. We have tried to give a broad overview of the science of prion diseases without going into the sort of detail that non-specialists might find intimidating. Some chapters will be more difficult than others for the non-specialist but we urge them to persevere; their appreciation of the nature of these diseases will be enhanced if they do. On the other hand, we hope that those working in the field will accept that our account is written for a general readership and will not be too critical if we have not dealt with issues of special interest to them in the way they would have preferred. We make no apology for concentrating on the 'protein only' hypothesis of prion diseases; we subscribe to the hypothesis. Although there are other views of which we make mention from time to time, especially in the suggested reading sections, we feel that a comprehensive evaluation of these other views would make another book, written, perhaps, by someone who supports them.

We offer our thanks to our friends, Robert Fishwick, Tony Palmer, and Judith Denton, who, between them, have read the complete book, and who have made many helpful comments.

Finally, we would like to remember our friend and colleague, Leo Duchen, who died in 1996. For a number of years, Leo was Professor of Neuropathology at the National Hospital for Neurology and Neurosurgery and the Institute of Neurology in London. We spent many long afternoons with him discussing the intricacies of neuropathology and the vanity of scientists, and eating Rich Tea biscuits.

Cambridge   R. M. R.
June 1997   H. F. B.

Contents

1 A peculiar protein   1
2 Concerning sheep   17
3 Kuru, a story of cannibalism   40
4 Creutzfeldt–Jakob disease, the emergence of
   a disease entity   65
5 In the laboratory   98
6 In the genes   114
7 Transgenes, transplants, and test tubes   134
8 Down on the farm: BSE   149
9 New variant CJD, a disease of old age
   in young people   179
10 What kind of disease is this?   207

Glossary   221

References   229

Recommended reading   240

Index   247

1

A peculiar protein

Human prion disease

The story of prion disease is a story of tragedies. Prion disease can affect both humans and animals and, when it does, it is invariably fatal, since it causes a neurodegenerative process in which the brain cells fall apart. There are no vaccines or medicines which will prevent disease and, apart from nursing care, no treatments to halt or slow its inevitable course. In comparison to other neurodegenerative diseases, such as Alzheimer's disease, Parkinson's disease, or motor neurone disease, its progression is usually alarmingly rapid. The patient's condition deteriorates almost daily as doctors attempt to make a diagnosis and the family struggles to accept what is happening. It can be so rapid that, initially, the illness may be misdiagnosed as 'stroke', and the patient may progress from health to death in a week or two. But the disease process actually bears a close resemblance to those of the much slower neurodegenerative diseases of old age, and some patients with prion disease may suffer mental and physical incapacity for many years.

Human prion disease can be caused in three different ways, known as *sporadic*, *familial*, or *acquired*. Each has its own peculiar tragedy. In most cases, where it is given the name sporadic Creutzfeldt–Jakob disease (CJD), it strikes in later middle age, completely 'out of the blue'. Sporadic CJD occurs throughout the world with an incidence of about one case per million of the population each year, and, although there is a very minor genetic contribution to the risk of developing disease, nothing is known to trigger it. It just seems to occur as an outrageous piece of bad luck which deterministic scientists, as well as people personally involved, find difficult to accept. None of the well-recognized precipitants of ill health, such as smoking, exposure to environmental pollutants, obesity, or stress, make any difference. Indeed, it can be argued that since CJD usually occurs in people of later middle age or older, a healthy lifestyle has a slightly risk-enhancing effect, since it ensures that the person lives further into the risk period.

In addition to those who develop prion disease sporadically, a tiny number of people, perhaps as few as 1 in 10 million of the population, carry an additional desperate secret. These unfortunate individuals harbour one of a number of specific genetic mutations which ensures that they will inevitably develop prion disease in the long term. They may be stricken while as young as 30, or the prospect of disease may hang over them, like the sword of Damocles, until they are nearly 70. The genetic forms of the disease have slightly different clinical and pathological features, depending on the precise gene mutation, and this will be discussed in later chapters. The different forms are described as familial CJD, Gerstmann–Sträussler–Scheinker disease (GSS), fatal familial insomnia (FFI), or, when the disease seems to fit none of these categories precisely, atypical prion disease (APD). These mutations illustrate the way in which evolution works in general. Genes only survive if the creatures in which they exist also survive to produce offspring which carry these genes. This ensures that organisms become ever more 'adapted' to the environment, that is, they become more and more sophisticated and successful. But a 'bad' gene, whose deleterious effect only becomes evident after the onset of reproductive ability, is not efficiently weeded out by evolutionary pressure, because the gene has already been passed on to some of the offspring before the organism dies. These deleterious genes, which evolution is unable to eliminate, have been referred to as 'senescence' genes, and the mutant genes which cause prion disease belong to this group. It is the continued existence of many such senescence genes, slowly contributing to the failure of many bodily organs, which means that death is inevitable for all of us.

In the late eighteenth and early nineteenth centuries in Britain, the Industrial Revolution heralded a marked change in domestic and social arrangements, especially amongst the poorer members of society. There was a major movement of people from the countryside to the increasingly overcrowded cities to join the workforce necessary to supply the burgeoning factories, the 'dark satanic mills' of William Blake. In the new economic system, in which it was essential to earn wages to procure the necessities of life, the poorhouse and the lunatic asylum were built to cope with those who were themselves unable to be economically productive and who were now deprived of family-based carers (Scull 1982). About this time there appeared the concept of 'hereditary insanity', which became a subject of fear and shame. Some of these patients, who in earlier times might have been cared for by their families in the villages but who, no doubt, ran the risk of being regarded with fear or ridicule, would have been suffering from Huntington's disease (another inherited neurodegenerative disease), young-onset familial Alzheimer's disease, or other, normally rare but incurable, diseases. Amongst these were the victims of familial prion disease for whom the asylum provided an austere but fundamentally well-meant protection from the social and economic pressures of Georgian and Victorian society.

Table 1.1 Prion diseases in humans

Sporadic disease (no known antecedent events)	Creutzfeldt–Jakob disease (CJD). Occurs worldwide with incidence of about 1 in a million
Acquired disease (acquired by contamination with infectious agent)	Kuru. Epidemic amongst the Foré people of Papua New Guinea Iatrogenic CJD New variant CJD. Thought to result from eating food contaminated with BSE agent.
Familial disease (genetically inherited)	Familial CJD. Accounts for about 10–15% of all CJD cases Gerstmann–Sträussler–Scheinker syndrome. Incidence about 1 in 10 million Fatal familial insomnia Atypical prion disease. Does not easily fit the various diagnostic criteria for prion disease

In present times, attitudes to mental and neurological illnesses have changed, but the problems facing families with inherited disease are still horrendous. For those with a family history of prion disease it is now possible, using modern techniques of genetic analysis, to predict with some certainty who will, and who will not, become ill. An 'at high risk' outcome provides no comfort; important life decisions such as whether to marry or to have children take on added dimensions. It might be thought that a 'not at risk' outcome would be welcomed with evident relief but experience now tells us that this is rarely true. Such an outcome often has profound psychological effects. A person, now told that he or she will escape the clutches of 'the family disease', may suffer from 'survivor guilt' and feel alienated from the rest of the family who remain bound together by their shared uncertainties. The risk status of fetuses can be established by prenatal testing, but this brings with it the moral, ethical, and religious colouring of a difficult decision as to whether or not to terminate an 'at risk' pregnancy.

Human prion disease was the first neurological disease for which the precise gene defect (rather than the approximate position of the defective gene on a particular chromosome) was established (Hsiao *et al.* 1989). The discovery of the gene for familial prion disease signalled the arrival of a new era in medical genetics in which it is possible to identify people who, if they live long enough, will eventually succumb to fatal neurological disease. The gene mutations involved in Huntington's disease, the inherited forms of Alzheimer's disease, motor neurone disease, spinocerebellar ataxia, and some other very rare, adult-onset, fatal diseases have now been found, and more will follow as science digs away at the molecular basis of these diseases. The ethical, psychological, and social difficulties which this wealth of predictive power produces are now quite widely discussed, although in many cases those who are the most vociferous are not those who are likely to be either directly or indirectly involved. As we shall see, prion disease has always generated deeply divisive arguments.

Some 50 years ago or more, in a remote part of the world which outsiders had scarcely visited, something terrible was happening. At first, just a few women and young children of the Foré-speaking tribe of the remote eastern highlands of Papua New Guinea showed signs of an unusual illness, which was to feature importantly in future years. They all died after a few months. To their relatives and friends, who called the illness 'kuru', it was obvious that these unfortunate people had been possessed by evil spirits. Sadly, and puzzlingly, some years later these same relatives and friends themselves succumbed to kuru. The tribes-people believed that witchcraft was at work. Indeed, according to the chronicles of Vincent Zigas, the young German doctor who brought kuru to the notice of Western medicine, these highlanders of Papua New Guinea had no concept of death by 'natural causes' (Zigas 1990). To them all death was the result of sorcery, and on the death of a relative they immediately looked for the culprit on whom to exact the ultimate revenge, 'the tukabu'. However, no magic potions or vengeful actions could protect them from kuru and, as the years went by, the number of cases rose steadily until a substantial number of the whole population was affected. The victims were mainly, but not exclusively, women and children, and clear clusters of disease occurred both at specific times and amongst groups of relatives and friends. During the 1950s, kuru became the most common cause of death amongst young women, and doctors trained in Western medicine had nothing to offer which could affect the course of the illness.

The kuru epidemic provides a rather dramatic example of the third way in which people can become affected with prion disease, for kuru is indeed a prion disease. Despite its usual sporadic or genetic occurrence, prion disease is also transmissible in the sense that one person can pass it on to another. Strictly speaking, prion disease is not 'infectious' since this term describes diseases which can be caught by air-borne transfer of a micro-organism. Nor is it a contagious disease in which infection is passed from one person to another by skin contact. Most of those transmissible diseases which are neither infectious nor contagious are sexually transmitted or blood-borne, but this is not the case for prion disease. Prion disease is transmissible only when some tissue from an affected person or animal enters the body of another person, either by being eaten, or by some other process, for example surgery or injection, through which tissue is deposited directly within the body of another person. As a result of an interesting series of scientific observations, suggestions, and experiments involving researchers from the United States, Australia, and Europe, it was established in 1966 that kuru was a transmissible disease (Gajdusek *et al.* 1966).

How did it spread? Interest focused on the possibility that cannibalism had a part to play. An anthropologist, Robert Glasse, had suggested that ritual cannibalism of dead family members was a funerary practice which had been prevalent in Papua New Guinea since the beginning of this century, and argued that the consumption of kuru victims had fuelled the epidemic. However, serious discussion about cannibalism has always been fraught with difficulties. While some tribes-people were prepared to admit to cannibalism, there has always been the problem that information gathered from another culture may be subject to serious misinterpretation. Accounts of cannibalism are fairly common in anthropological literature about obscure ethnic groups, and are not unknown amongst Westerners in certain unusual circumstances. Frequently, though, these are accounts of events that happened just before the anthropologists arrived, or in the next valley, or in a group against whom the story teller had a long-standing animosity. So, there was always the possibility that the witnesses were trying to denigrate their enemy, impress the anthropologists, or were speaking metaphorically. Equally, research workers can be prone to the sort of vanity that leaves them victims of their own credulousness and naivety. The early study of kuru added fuel to another burning argument in sociology about the value of 'not quite eye-witness' accounts, especially where cannibalism was suspected (Arens 1979). Emotionally charged debates took place between those who held the view that it was not 'politically correct' to believe that another racial group was capable of behaviour, which in Western culture is regarded as particularly heinous, and those who took the opposing view, that it was wrong to dismiss the verbal evidence of another racial group as if it were less reliable than evidence from members of one's own culture. But no amount of arguing could alter the fact that several thousand people in Papua New Guinea died of kuru in the middle part of this century and that, when the area came under Australian governmental control, the number of cases of kuru began to drop year by year. As time went by fewer and fewer cases appeared, and such cases were in progressively older people, making it clear that these poor people were the 'tail end' of the kuru epidemic and had been incubating disease, sometimes for many years. For them, kuru was the long-term consequence of something that had happened before the region was administered from Australia. Later research was to reveal that this exotic disease was closely related to the rare and usually sporadic CJD in the West. As a result of a funerary practice, which, even if it did not include cannibalism, must have involved some form of personal contamination by the women who prepared the bodies of the dead, and who fed themselves and their children at the same time, the Foré tribe of Papua New Guinea instigated a form of self-inflicted genocide. But before we condemn this as something from which 'civilization' protects us, we should consider that we may also have made a similar mistake.

Alarm bells began to sound in Switzerland when doctors realized that two young patients who had died of CJD, had both undergone neurosurgery in the same hospital on the same day, almost 2 years earlier, as another patient who was diagnosed at that time as having CJD (Brown 1996). A coincidence like this does not happen by chance, especially in relation to a disease that is so rare that it affects only one in a million people each year. A further handful of similarly suspicious cases in the United States and the United Kingdom was a portent of something that was to shock the medical profession deeply. During the 1950s and 1960s, a way had been found to extract human growth hormone from the pituitary gland (which is attached to the brain inside the skull) collected during post-mortem examinations, and to use this hormone to treat people of short stature. For the most part this treatment benefited those young people with damage to their own pituitary gland, rather than patients with achondroplasia (the most familiar cause of limited growth) for whom the new preparation had nothing to offer. In some countries, treatment was made available to children who were just small for their age, but who had no specific medical condition. In the mid-1980s, when it became known that two or three young sufferers from CJD had all received a course of growth hormone injections several years earlier, there was much consternation within the medical profession. The possibility that pituitaries might have been collected from the tiny number of patients with CJD, and that as a consequence the growth hormone preparations might have been contaminated, had not really been taken into account. That infectivity could have survived the dilution and chemical procedures involved in the preparation of the hormone seemed most unlikely. Yet happen it did, and at the present time iatrogenic (literally, generated by the doctor) CJD, mainly resulting from hormone replacement treatments, constitutes a significant proportion of cases of prion disease in young people (Brown 1996). Several thousand youngsters around the world were treated with human growth hormone, and the spectre of an epidemic arising as a result continues to haunt us. Inevitably there have been accusations of negligence and counterclaims of misadventure which have been the subject of litigation. Thus, prion disease has joined a burgeoning list of medical mishaps for which groups of patients are seeking redress.

Animal prion diseases

Animals can suffer from prion diseases. Scrapie, a prion disease of sheep, has been known in Europe for at least two centuries. The disease has always been stigmatized, accompanied by fear and secrecy amongst sheep farmers, who have no wish to see the market value of animals from their flocks falling. Then came BSE—bovine spongiform encephalopathy (Wells and Wilesmith 1995). In economic terms BSE has been the most serious epidemic ever to have affected farm animals in the United Kingdom and, apart from the prospect of a common currency, it has been the most difficult problem ever faced by the European Community. The full cost of the epidemic cannot be calculated, but in terms of compensation and lost revenue alone, it already runs into billions of pounds. In the 10 years between 1986 (when it first appeared) and 1996, more than 160 000 British cattle died of BSE. According to a paper published in the journal, *Nature*, in mid-1996, in which the BSE epidemic was modelled mathematically, it has been estimated that a further 700 000 cattle were also infected, although they were not showing signs of disease when they were slaughtered, many for human consumption. This figure remains, of course, an estimate and is not proven. In 1996 and 1997, millions of cattle in the United Kingdom were slaughtered in the cull policies designed to hasten the end of the epidemic and to protect the public.

The reports, in 1996, of a new form of CJD has prompted the speculation that several young people may have died as a consequence of eating BSE-

Table 1.1 Prion diseases in animals

Scrapie	A rare endemic brain disease of sheep and goats
Transmissible mink encephalopathy (TME)	A disease of farmed mink, probably caused by feeding scrapie-contaminated meat
Chronic wasting disease (CWD)	A scrapid-like disease, of obscure origin, in wild and captive mule deer and Rocky Mountain elk
Bovine spongiform encephalopathy (BSE)	Epidemic disease in dairy cows, mainly in the UK, caused by feeding cows with feedstuff containing rendered remains of scrapie-affected sheep and BSE-affected cattle
Feline spongiform encephalopathy (FSE)	Disease seen in domestic cats, and in a few other cats, including puma, cheetah, and ocelot. Assumed to be caused by feeding BSE-infected material
Spongiform encephalopathy in other species	Identified in a number of zoo animals; for example, kudu, gemsbok, nyala, eland, Arabian oryx, and scimitar. Assumed to be caused by feeding BSE-infected material

contaminated food, perhaps many years earlier. If this is so, we must face the possibility that there could be a few more cases, or contemplate the unthinkable, that over the next 20 years we will see the emergence of a major epidemic affecting an incalculable number of people in Britain. This would be the greatest tragedy of all; but it remains possible that the new form of CJD in young people seen in Britain in the last 2 years is not connected with BSE. However, whatever the outcome, many thousands of farmers, farm labourers, abattoir workers, livestock dealers, meat processors, butchers, renderers, feedstuff manufacturers, and fertilizer producers, to name only those most directly affected, have lost their livelihoods.

The emergence of BSE has deeply shocked the public. The media have covered the issues extensively and have even, on occasion, invited the public to vote on the question of whether BSE is a risk to humans. It is as if they thought that public opinion might in some way alter the behaviour of the disease. Most people are all too tolerant of situations which may lead to death in the far distant future so long as they can maintain the delusion that they can deal with it later. People are much less tolerant of what they perceive as 'time-bomb' diseases—chemicals or radiation—whose presence is difficult to detect but which may wreak havoc without warning years later. Frequent catastrophes like road accidents seem to be much more acceptable than infrequent catastrophes. Perhaps there is a feeling that if a calamity is rare then a certain amount of effort could avoid it, whereas if a problem is widespread it is just the way things are. BSE, like nuclear radiation, has been placed firmly in the 'zero risk tolerance' category by most of the public, both in Britain and overseas. BSE has also undermined public confidence in the ability of the government to handle emergencies, and of the scientist to provide useful and rational guidance. This loss of trust may take years to rebuild.

Arguments about prion disease

The story of prion disease is also a story of arguments. If prion disease has generated legal, ethical, social, and personal dilemmas, it has also stimulated profound, long-lasting, and acrimonious debate amongst scientists. Cutting argument has exposed the scientific method as being not quite so high minded or rational as we might be led to believe. Why should the study of prion disease have caused so much trouble? The first, and simplest, answer is that prion disease can have three wholly separate causes, and, for each, the circumstances which lead to disease are wholly different. However, the diseases are related in that these circumstances converge on a common pathogenic mechanism. The disease is either *naturally sporadic, genetically determined*, or *acquired by contamination*, and these three aetiologies (causes) do not interact. This is not the case for other diseases, which may be the result of many interacting factors (for example smoking, high blood pressure, and a sedentary lifestyle combine to increase risk of heart attack). Any specific case of prion disease is either sporadic, genetic, or acquired in origin. This separateness only became explicit in the 1980s (Ridley *et al.* 1986). Before that time it was generally assumed, as it still is by some scientists, that any evidence about how a particular type of prion disease occurred was relevant to an understanding of all cases of prion disease. Thus the demonstration that kuru, CJD, and scrapie were all transmissible under experimental (and highly contrived) conditions led to the conclusion that all cases of prion disease occurring naturally in either people or animals must have been acquired by some form of contamination. Yet neurologists were unable to discover anything peculiar about the behaviour or occupations of patients with sporadic CJD. In addition, the existence of families with more than one case of a CJD-like illness was well known to neurologists, although this occurrence is so rare that most clinicians would not personally encounter such families during their entire career. It was unrealistic to suppose that these families were doing something that was even inadvertently cannibalistic. Scientists and clinicians have no difficulty accepting that there can be a number of different ways to catch a disease. For example, HIV, the human immunodeficiency virus which causes AIDS, can be transmitted sexually or through the use of blood products, as happened in the case of haemophiliacs treated with factor VIII. But for nearly 40 years the idea that prion disease might be acquired by contamination in some cases, but not in others, was scientifically unacceptable. Veterinarians, in particular, were determined that scrapie was an acquired disease, while other scientists argued equally strongly that much of the evidence about prion disease was incompatible with an acquired cause. So the debate went on. While scientists marshalled the evidence supporting one argument, they ignored the data they could not accommodate within that argument. Like novices trying to solve the puzzle of Rubik's cube, one single-coloured face of the cube could be constructed if the colours of the other faces were ignored. But it is not possible to solve Rubik's cube by doing one face at a time. A wider strategy is required, in which partially completed faces have to be sacrificed, in order to produce an accumulation of order which eventually leads to all the faces falling into place at once. The reluctance of scientists to loosen up on what they thought they knew impeded their understanding of the aetiology of prion disease.

Many of the great debates of science have been solved, not by one side being proved right and the other wrong, but by the realization that a better truth lies outside the immediate preoccupations of the protagonists. In physics, the debate about whether subatomic particles behave like 'waves' or 'billiard balls' has been resolved by the acceptance that both models have explanatory power, rather than by arguing that evidence in favour of one model is evidence against another model. In the nature/nurture debate about human behaviour, especially intelligence, neither side has won. However, the fire has gone out of the debate because modern molecular analysis has demonstrated beyond all reasonable doubt that genetics makes a major contribution to most aspects of the human condition, including physical attributes, behaviour, and mental illness. But, equally, the involvement of environmental factors in mental as well as physical conditions in later life is becoming established by epidemiological analysis. So, the transmissibility of prion disease does not negate the existence of spontaneous generation of disease in both sporadic and familial cases. A full understanding of prion disease must take all aetiologies into account.

The right framework

The second reason why prion disease research has caused so much confusion is that for many years there was no theoretical framework into which it could easily be fitted. Much twentieth century scientific investigation has taken place within a useful framework—we are thinking, for example, of the micro-organism theory of infection, the nucleic acid theory of genetic inheritance, or the antibody theory of immunity. Much of the research on prion disease was done against no clear theoretical background, or within an established framework that turned out to be inappropriate. This is a salutary lesson, since it indicates that well-meaning and conscientious scientists can work for years, accumulating enough positive evidence to keep their beliefs intact, when in fact they have got hold of completely the wrong end of the stick. It has been remarked that a theory, however wrong, rarely dies before its author. We may wonder why astronomers and mathematicians could work for a thousand years plotting the heavenly movements of celestial bodies, labouring all the time under the certain knowledge that the sun rotated around the earth. Or we may smile at the toiling alchemist, who tried for decades to change base metal into gold, when no modern chemist has the slightest doubt that this is impossible. For 30 years the major research effort in the spongiform encephalopathies consisted of a search for the virus or other micro-organism which, it was thought, *must* have been responsible for the transmissibility of these diseases, despite growing evidence that no such organism exists. Most scientists have now abandoned the search, but a few cling to the concept that these diseases are caused by a virus and continue to present data which they think support the existence of an independent infectious agent.

According to the philosopher Thomas Kuhn, science progresses by a series of revolutions or 'paradigm shifts' (Kuhn 1962). An interesting phenomenon may emerge from collected data. Attempts at an explanation lead to the development of a theoretical framework into which more data are patiently fitted. But the proper method of science is not to acquire data whose only use is to support a theory indefinitely. Rather it is to think of experiments that can prove that the theory is wrong if it is wrong (Popper 1959). In other words it is the job of a good scientist to generate 'testable hypotheses' based on the theory and to be able to falsify them. This second phase of data collection and hypothesis testing is 'normal science', and many scientists will spend their entire career working in this 'normal' mode. Eventually the theory collapses amidst consternation, and a period of furious dissent and confusion follows until another, better, theoretical framework emerges. But science, like history, is written by the victors, and one might be forgiven for thinking that a scientific 'breakthrough' is a moment of insight, certainty, and happiness. In fact, the emergence of a radical new theory in science is perhaps the most frightening as well as the most exciting event in a scientist's career. As in a political *coup d'état,* the proponent risks all. If his new ideas are disproved by evidence, or his fellow scientists reject them as seriously flawed, his career in science may be jeopardized. Colleagues may also feel threatened in the face of such changes in approach, and may be aggressive. If they nail their colours to the new theory, they lose the comfort of the old framework and risk ridicule if the theory falls under the weight of the evidence, which others will undoubtedly try to muster. But if they remain loyal to the old ways they may end up as unimaginative 'has beens' whose work is relegated to the dusty shelves at the back of the library.

In 1982, Stan Prusiner, a neurologist and biochemist at the University of California in San Francisco, published a paper in the journal, *Science,* in which he proposed that the transmissible agent of the spongiform encephalopathies was not an organism similar to a virus, but rather that it was radically different from any other infectious particle and consisted (probably entirely) of an abnormal protein (Prusiner 1982). This he christened the 'prion', a name constructed from '*proteinaceous infectious particle*'. This proposition has been widely misinterpreted as contravening the central dogma of molecular biology, which holds that nucleic acid *alone* has the power of duplicating itself and contains the information that determines the structure of proteins. Prusiner argued that a protein could be 'infectious', which seemed to imply the ability to duplicate itself in the *absence* of DNA, and for this he was ridiculed. Such a contravention could be likened to the effect that Darwin's presentation of his theory of evolution and the origin of the human species had on the creationists of his time. In fact the 'prion hypothesis', as it is now called, in no way conflicts with the central dogma. What it does do is to shift the central dogma from its all powerful position by arguing that nucleic acid is not the only form of stored, heritable, or replicable information in biological systems. The role of the prion hypothesis is perhaps more like that of the theory of relativity which, while not refuting Newtonian physics, does indicate that such a theory is limited in its applicability.

Working with prion disease

Not only the lack of an appropriate theoretical framework hampered the unravelling of the complexities of prion disease; progress was also seriously impeded by difficulties in experimental practicality. The most important prion disease for most of this century, in terms of numbers of victims and economic costs, has been scrapie in sheep. But the inconvenience of working with sheep was a major problem for early researchers, since most experiments on this disease require the use of large numbers of animals. This problem was solved in the early 1960s when scientists demonstrated that sheep scrapie could be transmitted to mice by intracerebral injection; this 'mouse-adapted scrapie' could then be studied within the comfort of a laboratory. However, serious difficulties have arisen because the behaviour of this 'artificial' disease has not always paralleled the natural disease in sheep. The detection and quantification of infective 'agent' in tissue presented another difficulty. Most researchers could expect to find the result of an experiment (known as the dependent variable, the thing that varies according to what you have done) in a biochemical reaction in a test tube, or as something that could be viewed down the microscope. In scrapie research the only way to detect the presence of the infectious agent in tissue was to inject it into the brain of an animal—usually a laboratory mouse or hamster—and then wait up to a year to see whether the animal became sick.

During the 1980s laboratories throughout the world collaborated in trying to identify the infectious agent in prion diseases. The homogenized (blended) brains of infected hamsters were fractionated (separated) into a number of different components, in an attempt to concentrate the infectivity within one component. The most infectious fraction was found to contain large amounts of a particular protein that was not destroyed by enzymes that normally break down proteins (proteolytic enzymes). This protein (subsequently christened prion protein, or PrP, by Stan Prusiner) was not found when normal, uninfected, hamster brain was subjected to the same processing. Proteins are made of strings of amino acids, and the protein in infected brain was identical in its sequence of amino acids (known as its primary structure) to a protein that was present in equal quantities in infected and uninfected brain tissue, but which was readily broken down by proteolytic enzymes. Therefore there were two forms of the same protein. The form found only in infected brain was subsequently called PrP^{sc} (where ^{sc} stands for scrapie) and that found in both infected and uninfected brain was called PrP^{c} (where ^{c} stands for cellular).

Earlier, Pat Merz in New York had discovered that when extracts of brain tissue from scrapie-affected animals were examined in an electron microscope, small rod-like structures could be seen. These structures, which she called 'scrapie-associated fibrils' or SAFs, are composed of a partially broken down PrP^{sc}. SAFs can sometimes coalesce in the test tube to form insoluble lumps, known as 'amyloid'. The term amyloid is used to describe a particular state of matter, like 'glue', or 'jelly', or 'polymer'. Although SAFs are 'artificial' structures made by chemical processing of brain extracts in the test tube, similar deposits of prion protein amyloid are sometimes seen under the microscope in brain sections. Many proteins are sticky or lumpy and their molecules bind to each other to form normal amyloid substances, such as silk and cobweb. But such a chemical capability can go wrong and the accumulation of abnormal amyloids that cause tissue damage are pathological features of many diseases. The most familiar of these is Alzheimer's disease, in which deposits of another type of amyloid (called β-amyloid) are found throughout the brain. Although the preparation of SAFs can be used as a diagnostic test for prion disease when levels of infectivity are fairly high, SAFs are not themselves the infectious agent and do not exist in the brain of the affected animal. Rather, they are created from the complete prion protein by the harsh biochemical techniques that are used in the test-tube to prepare the material for microscopical analysis. Although PrP-amyloid is deposited in the form of 'plaques' in the brain in some cases of prion disease but not in others, there seems to be an inverse relationship between the amount of PrP-amyloid and the amount of infectivity in brain tissue samples.

What does the abnormal form of prion protein (PrP^{sc}) have to do with the infectious agent? The answer seems to lie in the fact that PrP^{sc} is the only substance consistently and exclusively found in conjunction with infectivity. Could they be one and the same thing? Because it is made and broken down rapidly, the amount of PrP^{c} in the brain does not change when an animal becomes infected with prion disease. However, the level of PrP^{sc} does rise during the incubation period of the disease because it is never broken down, and therefore accumulates in the tissue. In experiments in which an animal of one species (for example, a mouse) developed disease after being injected with brain tissue from an affected animal of another species (for example, a hamster), the PrP^{sc} in the mouse was 'mouse-made' protein not 'hamster-made' protein. This made it clear that PrP^{sc} did not itself *replicate*, which, as we have said, would have been heretical for biologists. But it did seem that a unique interaction was taking place in which the PrP^{sc} from the hamster was in some way persuading the normal

PrP^c of the mouse to change into the abnormal, disease-associated PrP^{sc} form. It is now widely accepted that this is the basis of the transmissibility of prion disease, both in laboratory experiments and in naturally occurring circumstances, such as those leading to kuru, iatrogenic CJD, and BSE.

The next compelling piece of evidence that set the prion protein at centre stage came from the study of that tiny number of families affected with more than one case of prion disease. Genetic analysis of the affected members of the family indicated that one of the two copies of the PrP gene that they carry contained a very rare mutation which was not found in the rest of the population. Using genetic engineering techniques, scientists in Prusiner's laboratory modified the DNA in mice so that these animals carried a number of copies of the PrP gene containing a mutation equivalent to that found in the PrP gene in these families. These genetically modified mice spontaneously developed prion disease in adulthood. The slightly different PrP protein produced by these mutant PrP genes seemed to change *spontaneously* from PrP^c to PrP^{sc} and to precipitate the disease in mice that had not encountered any PrP^{sc} from elsewhere. The rare, familial occurrence of the disease in humans is explained in the same way.

Murphy's law states that 'where something can go wrong, it will', and this is very much the case in biology. Although evolution has moulded the possible into the advantageous, the disadvantageous will always be lurking in the shadows of existence. The need for proteins to form larger structures makes the three-dimensional shape of proteins very important. PrP^c and PrP^{sc} have different shapes. The ability of proteins to take on different shapes means that sometimes this process will happen when it should not. Thus it seems that PrP^c sometimes converts to PrP^{sc} without a specific precipitating event, leading to the occurrence of sporadic prion disease. Evolution has ensured that the normal form of PrP is extremely unlikely to undergo these changes and that, when it does, it is as part of the senescence process, after the age at which the animal has reproduced. But new mutations in the PrP gene will occur from time to time. If mutations produced a prion protein that immediately took on the PrP^{sc} form, the effects would be lethal before birth and they would never be detected. But where the change from PrP^c to PrP^{sc} is delayed until adulthood, the gene will survive, be passed on to any offspring and, ultimately, contribute to the burden of adult-onset genetic disease.

We have included this very brief overview of the rest of the book and introduction to the biochemistry of prion disease in order to help the reader anticipate how the many facets of prion disease will come together. The paradox of prion disease is not entirely resolved, but we hope that in the following chapters we will be able to give an account of how we have come to know what we do know, and what false trails have beset an understanding of this disease.

2

Concerning sheep

The early reports of scrapie

Some years ago 'Call my bluff' was a popular game show on British television. Members of one team had to provide imaginative definitions of some very strange words, and those of the opposing team then had to guess which was the correct definition and which were just too ridiculous to be true. The celebrity tried valiantly to convince her opponents that 'scrapie' was 'a dementing illness of middle-aged sheep'. Of course, no one believed her, the mere suggestion that any such illness could exist being greeted with hoots of derision!

Until the end of the 1960s scrapie was an arcane subject, of obsessive interest to a small number of veterinarians and animal pathologists, but largely ignored by other scientists. It was recognized as a 'peculiar' disease and horrendously difficult to research. Times have changed, and there can now be few people in Britain who have not heard of scrapie in connection with BSE. Faced, in 1986, with the realization that a new spongiform encephalopathy was occurring in British cattle, scientists at the Central Veterinary Laboratory in Surrey turned at first to the only other spongiform encephalopathy in farm animals, that is, scrapie, for clues to both the origin and the likely future occurrence of BSE. We think that this was the best that they could have done at the time, although they were aware that there were certain disadvantages to this approach. Prior to the emergence of BSE, scrapie research in Britain had been in decline for some years, and a number of the scientists who had been the most knowledgeable about the disease in sheep had retired or died. Much of what was known about scrapie was based on experiments in which large numbers of sheep had to be maintained for many years. Such experiments could not easily be repeated, so data were not often subject to the degree of replication and confirmation that is common in most areas of science. We think that very little knowledge about sheep scrapie was firmly established by 1986 and that not a great deal more is known now. Scrapie is endemic in sheep, occurring at a low level in many parts of the world, while, in the late 1980s, it was clear that BSE was a very rapidly growing epidemic. None the less, research into prion disease began with research on scrapie and it is important to understand the background from which scrapie arose. The history of scrapie was researched and recorded in great detail by Herbert B. Parry (known as James!), but his sudden death in 1980 prevented him from writing his account, which he thought might have amounted to 750 000 words. His friend, David Oppenheimer, collated what data he could from the huge collection of papers left by Parry, publishing them in a small volume entitled *Scrapie disease in sheep* (Parry 1983). We hope to show you that what started as the study of a few mangy sheep with a nervous itch has indeed led to a revolution in biology.

The original sheep of Britain were small, often brown, horned varieties which we could call 'Celtic'. Larger, white, often hornless, 'Roman' sheep from the continent were introduced during the time of the Roman occupation. The extent of the Roman Empire, encompassing as it did large parts of Europe, the Middle East, and North Africa, provided widespread opportunities for trade and transportation, and small numbers of Asiatic and North African breeds of sheep were imported into Britain, increasing the genetic diversity. The wool trade was of major economic importance in the Middle Ages, especially for the land-owning monasteries, and by the fourteenth century there were between 15 and 18 million sheep (but only 4 million people) in Britain. In comparison, there are now more than 50 million people and about 40 million sheep. The hardiness of sheep meant that they could be left to graze on non-arable ground without much human interference. Such sheep farming did not change much until the eighteenth century, when new methods of breed improvement were adopted. Large numbers of merino sheep, with a particularly fine wool, were introduced from Spain, and breeders were keen to cross this valuable asset with the hardiness of indigenous 'Celtic' and 'Roman' sheep. It was at this point that scrapie, variously described as 'rubbers', 'cuddytrot', 'euky pine', 'goggles', and 'scratchie', but readily recognizable from descriptions of the clinical signs, was reported throughout Britain. The disease also appeared in continental Europe, where it was known as '*Traberkrankheit*' or '*Gnubberk-rankheit*' in Germany, and as '*la tremblante*' or '*la maladie folle*' in France. The Journal of the House of Commons (1754–55) records complaints from country squires that the disease, which it was thought might be either hereditary or infectious, was being spread by sheep dealers who were mixing 'tainted' with 'untainted' stock. After much deliberation, no action was taken, and nearly 250 years later, the British government was still debating whether to attempt to eradicate scrapie by treating genetic or infectious aspects of the disease.

It is not clear whether it was the importation of merino sheep which introduced the disease into Britain, or whether the increase in scrapie was due solely to subsequent attempts to manipulate the quality of sheep by in-breeding. During the nineteenth century many flocks of merino sheep were exported from Spain to Australia, New Zealand, and South America, where scrapie is not seen. But it seems that even by the eighteenth century, merino sheep, which were kept by isolated, nomadic groups in Spain, were becoming separated into different sub-breeds. The merinos which came to Europe and which were associated with the subsequent appearance of scrapie were mainly of the 'Escorial' type, whereas those animals which were sent to the antipodes were mainly of the 'Negretti' variety. It is probable that millions of sheep are descended from single flocks which were moved from one region to another. These historical 'bottlenecks' can lead to the segregation of genetic traits between animals of apparently the same breed or stock.

During the early part of the eighteenth century, attempts to improve sheep stock included breeding 'in-and-in', that is, by mating fathers with daughters and sons with mothers, the results of which were catastrophic. Within 20 years scrapie was prevalent throughout lowland Britain, with many flocks losing more than 10 per cent of the ewes each year. Since sheep farming has always been a low-profit enterprise, such losses completely wiped out any financial gain and the flocks were destroyed. Scrapie does not become apparent until sheep are 3–5 years old, by which age ewes may have had some offspring, and stud rams may have served hundreds of ewes. Lambs which were, therefore, likely to be genetically susceptible to scrapie were often sold on, either innocently or as an attempt to recoup some of the losses resulting from the high levels of scrapie in the flock, and so the disease persisted. For breeding purposes, the choice of sheep which were susceptible to scrapie may not have been just a matter of bad luck. In the twentieth century, Steele (1964) reported that those Suffolk rams which subsequently succumbed to scrapie were the 'best' rams in adolescence, and were, therefore, likely to be selected for breeding. Such rams might have been chosen specifically to sire lambs for slaughter before 18 months of age, since the disease would not be apparent at that age and the meat was judged to be particularly desirable by butchers (Parry 1983). Provided none of the ewe lambs was retained for breeding, this would be commercially advantageous to the ewe-flock owner, and it would encourage the stud-flock owner to keep some scrapie in his flock.

The demonstration that scrapie is transmissible

The risk, which in-breeding produced, of sheep developing all manner of diseases and bad traits led, in the nineteenth century, to less intensive efforts at improving stock. Shepherds traced and killed the offspring of scrapie-affected animals, and the occurrence of scrapie seems to have declined dramatically until it was described as 'an obscure disease of sheep' (Stockman 1913). Then, in 1936, French scientists Cuillé and Chelle announced that they had transmitted scrapie to a healthy sheep by intraocular injection (that is, within the eye under general anaesthetic) of spinal cord tissue taken from an affected sheep (Cuillé and Chelle 1936). This, in itself, might not have been taken too seriously, since the time between injection and sickness was about 18 months, during which the recipient animal remained well. Eighteen months seemed in those days to have been too long for there to have been any causal connection. But this experiment was soon followed by an 'accidental experiment' carried out in Scotland by a veterinarian, W. S. Gordon. In the late 1930s he was working on the development of a vaccine against louping-ill, another serious disease of sheep (Palmer 1959). The vaccine he produced was made from tissues, including brain and spleen, from sheep already affected with louping-ill. These tissue preparations were treated with formalin in order to inactivate the virus which causes louping-ill, and injected into sheep, with the expectation that the inoculated animals would become immune to the virus. Unfortunately, as is now well known, the transmissible agent in scrapie is not destroyed by formalin. One batch of vaccine was made from tissues from a group of sheep, some of which were the offspring of ewes which later died of scrapie. Eighteen thousand sheep were inoculated with vaccine from this batch, and 2–3 years later it was recorded that up to 35 per cent of the animals in the vaccinated flocks developed scrapie, the previous incidence of the disease in these flocks having not been commercially noteworthy. The true transmission rate in these flocks was probably higher than was indicated by the number of sick animals, because older animals would have died or been sold before they showed symptoms of disease. There were, however, different disease rates in different flocks, indicating that there might be a genetic component to susceptibility to infection from an outside source. Gordon then set up an experiment to confirm his worst fear, that he had been responsible for a massive increase in the level of scrapie in these flocks. He injected 788 sheep with tissue from scrapie-infected animals. Sixty per cent of those animals receiving injections directly into the brain (intracerebrally) developed scrapie, while 30 per cent of those receiving injections under the skin (subcutaneously) became sick. In another experiment more than 1000 sheep of 24 different breeds were injected with brain tissue, all on the same day by the same people (Pattison 1992), so that the incidence in different breeds and stock lines could be determined. They did big experiments in those days! After several years it turned out that some breeds were much more susceptible than others, and that some breeds seemed to be totally resistant. Even in the most susceptible breeds a substantial majority of animals did not become sick. As we will explain later in this chapter, the past few years have seen a growing understanding of the precise genetic basis of the different sensitivities of different breeds. However, at the time of these early large-scale experiments, the demonstration that scrapie could be so readily transmitted from affected to unaffected animals (even if by highly contrived means) blinded scientists to the importance of genetics in the occurrence of this disease, and much of the historical evidence and knowledge of the sheep breeders was ignored.

The work of Gordon and his colleagues allowed the characteristics of 'experimental' scrapie to be studied in detail and to be compared to those of naturally occurring or 'field' cases. The disease occurs naturally in sheep, usually between the ages of 3 and 5 years, with a few cases occurring in animals which live to be 6 or 7 years old. By experimental transmission, the incubation period (from injection to onset of illness) varies from about 9 months to 3 years. The shortest incubation times are seen when brain tissue (rather than tissue from other, peripheral, parts of the body) is used as a source of infectious material, when large amounts of such tissue are used, and when the route of infection is intracerebral rather than subcutaneous. Thus, if field cases of scrapie occur because lambs are becoming infected, and if it is assumed that infection occurs shortly after the lambs are born, the late age at onset of disease could reflect a relatively inefficient mode of transmission of small amounts of infectivity. Or it could indicate that the natural disease has a very different cause (aetiology) from the experimentally transmitted cases. Curiously, the brain neuropathology in experimentally induced scrapie is said to be more pronounced than that seen in the naturally occurring disease, suggesting that there may be important differences between these two conditions, even though one is induced by using tissue from the other.

Recognizing sheep with scrapie

In scrapie disease, onset is slow, with only minor changes in demeanour occurring at first. A sheep may become 'jittery', or at odds with its fellows, standing separately from others when the others are lying, facing in the opposite direction from the rest of the flock, and so on. Such sheep appear anxious or agitated, and panic when attempts are made to drive them with sheepdogs. Two main forms of the disease have been described—'scratching', where the animal persistently rubs or scratches at parts of the skin which seem to itch, and 'nervous', where the animal seems to be particularly sensitive to noises or movements around it. However, our colleague, Tony Palmer, points out that this distinction is somewhat artificial, and that there is marked overlap in clinical presentation between these two forms. People familiar with scrapie are fond of saying that one should 'note the dull, vacant expression' on the faces of some affected sheep, but perhaps the rest of us may be forgiven for wondering in what way this expression differs from that of normal sheep. In fact, the animal is more likely to have an anxious expression on its face. Affected animals go on to develop neurological signs, which include an unsteadiness of the back legs, tremor, prolonged bouts of rubbing or scratching of parts of the body until the wool and sometimes the skin is lost, and a loss of general condition and weight (despite having a voracious appetite). They also walk with the high-stepping, trotting gait known as the 'cuddytrot'. Finally, they become incapacitated and are either destroyed by the farmer or fall down and die in the field. Scrapie cases can, however, vary considerably in their presentation, so that some sheep are found moribund without previous signs being noted, while for others the signs are so mild and non-specific that they may be regarded as being just 'poor stock' and disposed of. Since individual sheep are not of great value, the farmer may find it cheaper to kill a sheep than to pay a veterinarian to make it better, irrespective of the illness. Scrapie is less likely to be noticed in highland sheep, which are out of sight of their owners for much of the year, than in those sheep that live on lowland pastures. The variability in the signs of scrapie, and in the conditions under which sheep are kept, makes the collection of data on natural scrapie very difficult.

The neuropathology seen in the brains of sheep with scrapie differs somewhat between animals, but it includes certain essential features. Three areas of the brain are particularly affected: the most posterior part of the brain including the *cerebellum*, which controls, amongst other things, balance and the ability to walk without staggering or falling; the *brainstem*, which maintains levels of arousal; and the *hypothalamus*, that part of the brain which interacts with the pituitary gland (situated on the base of the brain) and which controls hormone secretion, eating behaviour, and many aspects of energy metabolism. The tissue damage in these three brain areas is responsible for the staggering gait, the hyperactivity and general nervousness, and the changes in appetite and physical condition of sheep with scrapie.

Within the affected areas of the brain, the main neuropathological feature is a loss of nerve cells (neurones), but without the signs of inflammation that would be expected in a viral encephalitis. A much discussed feature in the early work was the 'neuronal vacuolation'. Neuronal vacuolation is the term used to describe the formation of small bubbles within neurones, visible under a high-power microscope. This vacuolation is, however, usually accompanied by larger holes (spongiform change) which appear within the substance of the brain, and which give the brain tissue the appearance of a sponge under a low-power microscope. A milder form of vacuolation in brain tissue, caused by the death of neurones, can be seen in some rapidly progressive cases of a variety of neurodegenerative disease (Ironside 1996a). This non-specific change is sometimes referred to as 'status spongiosus'. The term spongiform encephalopathy is reserved for the very marked spongiform change accompanied by neuronal vacuolation seen exclusively in prion disease. Having asked many neuropathologists to explain to us exactly how they tell the difference between spongiform encephalopathy and status spongiosus, the answer has usually been that 'spongiform encephalopathy has a certain feel about it'! It seems to have something to do with the texture of the holes and their usual distribution in grey matter (the parts of the brain composed mainly of nerve cells) rather than in white matter (the parts of the brain containing many fibre tracts). When spongiform encephalopathy is present, it is diagnostic of prion disease. But sometimes spongiform encephalopathy is absent, or very minimal, making diagnosis of prion disease by neuropathological examination much more difficult. Although there are many features of prion disease which, when present, are highly suggestive or even definitive of prion disease, there are no features which are present in every case. Diagnosis may depend, therefore, on finding one or two features that are *typical* of prion disease. Such uncertainty is not confined to the prion diseases, and makes diagnosis a difficult matter for many diseases.

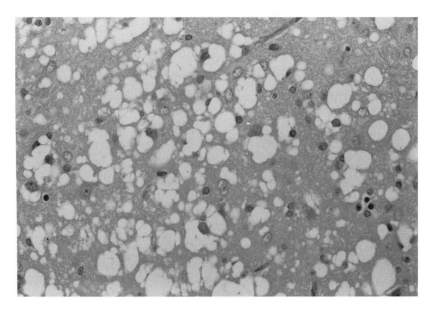

Fig. 2.1 Spongiform change in the brain of an animal with prion disease. The tissue contains many small bubble-like structures, called vacuoles, which gives the brain sections their spongy appearance under the microscope. (Photograph by G. A. H. Wells; magnification ∼ 400)

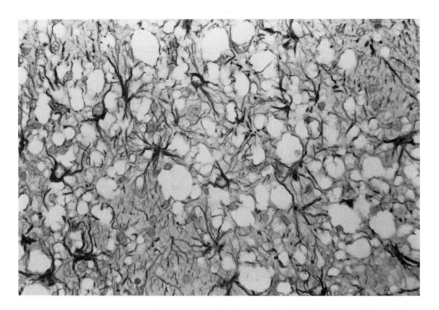

Fig. 2.2 This section from the brain of a patient with prion disease has been specifically stained to showed the spidery astrocytes which proliferate in response to neurodegeneration (magnification ∼ 400). The spongiform change in this brain can also be seen. (Photograph by L. W. Duchen.)

May sheep safely graze?

This was the first question asked about scrapie in the eighteenth century, and it will probably not be answered until the beginning of the next century. Many scientific accounts state baldly that sheep catch scrapie from one another by 'lateral transmission', that is, either by direct contact or by grazing the same pasture. Such statements imply that lateral transmission is so well accepted by the scientific community that no supporting evidence is required. We have been unable to find any original data that convinces us that lateral transmission occurs under natural conditions. There are numerous anecdotal reports that scrapie appeared suddenly in a group of sheep where it was previously unknown, but, as we shall see, such 'outbreaks' of scrapie are explained just as well by the hypothesis that natural scrapie may be a genetic disease as by the idea that sheep can catch scrapie from each other. Just because sheep come from a scrapie-free *flock* does not mean that they come from scrapie-free *stock*. Most commercial flocks are composed almost entirely of ewes and their lambs, the lambs being sold for meat when only a few months old. The few rams needed to serve the flock are frequently bought in and, while it may be possible to establish where such a purchased ram was born, the origin of *its* parental ram may be very obscure. For some reason the *paternal* ancestors of scrapie-affected sheep never seem to be blamed for introducing the disease.

Scrapie is sometimes said to have appeared in sheep which have been moved from a scrapie-free area to an area where scrapie was already occurring. But could this not mean that those working in the area to which the sheep had been moved were better at recognizing scrapie than those in the area from which the sheep had come? In judging whether this is plausible it would be helpful to know just how common scrapie is, and this turns out to be surprisingly difficult to determine. The majority of sheep farmers in Britain do not admit to ever having seen a case of scrapie in their flocks, and, where the disease does occur, usually no more than 1 or 2 per cent of sheep are affected in any one year (Morgan *et al.* 1990). There are exceptions to this, for example, in research institutes where sheep are bred for high susceptibility to disease, and in some unusual 'outbreaks'. In Iceland, scrapie was at one time so common that as many as 20 per cent of a flock could die of the disease in a year (Sigurdarson 1991).

Veterinarian Jim Hourrigan and his colleagues, based at the large sheep station at Mission, Texas, have studied the spread of scrapie throughout America (Hourrigan *et al.* 1979). It is clear that the disease was introduced with the importation from Britain of flocks of mainly Suffolk sheep, and that it spread rapidly during the first half of the twentieth century. Wherever these apparently healthy sheep or their offspring were moved, the disease was likely to follow. But whether the sheep were providing genetic susceptibility, or the infectious agent, or indeed both, cannot be determined from these observations. The fact that scrapie could arise in a flock, following the introduction of sheep which did not themselves develop scrapie, led to the concept of the 'asymptomatic carrier state', in which animals could carry the illness for all their life, but never show symptoms. However, to suppose that sheep with no signs of scrapie are, none the less, capable of carrying scrapie indefinitely seems to us unwarranted. There are other explanations for the sudden appearance of disease in a healthy flock. If scrapie were a recessive disease (in which both copies of one gene—remember, a copy of each gene is inherited from each parent—have to be defective for disease to appear), one would expect that sheep carrying only one defective copy of the gene would not themselves be ill. If they were mated with a new sheep that also carried one defective copy of this gene, some of the offspring would inherit a defective copy from both parents and disease would appear in the flock.

The evidence that lateral transmission occurred amongst the sheep and goats born at Mission includes the claim that the longer the lambs were left within a 'contaminated' environment (that is, in contact with affected animals) before they were removed, the more likely they were to develop scrapie themselves in later life. This, it was suggested, meant that these lambs became infected during the first few months of life. However, having examined the data published by Hourrigan and colleagues, we cannot see how the 'percentage of animals' they quote as being affected is derived from the actual number of animals documented. They also claimed that lateral transmission of disease occurred between sheep with scrapie and some of the *offspring* of '*previously unexposed goats*'. But some of these '*unexposed goats*' themselves had scrapie. So, where did they get it from? We have spent many years trying to understand the literature on the occurrence of scrapie in sheep and goats, particularly with an eye on the possibility of the occurrence of lateral transmission, and have come to the conclusion that most of the work was done without adequate controls, or on small numbers of animals of uncertain origin, or was so badly written up that it is now uninterpretable.

Data such as these provided the 'facts' about scrapie which underpinned decision making at the beginning of the BSE epidemic. It is disappointing that while several millions of pounds have been spent on research into BSE, investment in understanding naturally occurring scrapie in sheep has been minimal. Since scrapie was made a notifiable disease in the United Kingdom in 1993 the number of cases being reported is now lower than the number of cases collected informally for research purposes in 1992, suggesting that the disease has gone 'underground' and that the surveillance system is largely ineffectual.

An early observation in investigations of the lateral transmission of scrapie was that disease was never seen to pass to another sheep from sheep *experimentally* infected with scrapie, and that stories of lateral transmission were always associated with natural outbreaks of scrapie. It is possible that in field conditions it is especially difficult to be sure that sheep introduced into an affected flock really did come from a scrapie-free background; this may be less of a problem in carefully set up experiments. Another possibility is that in commercial flocks, in which the lateral spread of naturally occurring disease was said to have occurred, flock members were related to each other (sheep born in one year may all share one parental ram). In such circumstances the spread of disease by lateral transmission or genetic inheritance could not be distinguished.

Perhaps there was something about natural cases of scrapie which did not apply to experimentally infected sheep. For example, commercial flocks contained pregnant sheep and lambs, while experimentally infected sheep were usually not allowed to breed. Iain Pattison and his colleagues at Compton Research Station in Berkshire fed 12 sheep and 18 goats with the placenta and fetal membranes collected from scrapie-affected sheep. The same numbers of sheep and goats were injected intracerebrally with inoculum (homogenate) prepared from placental tissue. Over the following 2–3 years, scrapie developed in five of the sheep and three of the goats fed placental material, and in four of the sheep and one of the goats that received intracerebral injections. However, these experiments were done on only a handful of sheep, unlike the experiments which Iain Pattison did together with W. S. Gordon using hundreds of sheep. No 'control' animals were fed on placenta from unaffected sheep or fed on other tissues, or not fed on anything special at all. Indeed, the experiment was not properly finished and not all the data were published since 24 of the 36 goats went missing from the literature. This is very unfortunate because this experiment has been interpreted as demonstrating that scrapie is passed from ewe to lamb (a process known as maternal transmission), and that maternal transmission explains the occurrence of most cases of natural scrapie. Maternal transmission became a central tenet of scrapie epidemiology, unchallenged until 1995, and, in our view, has caused much confusion in the world of BSE (Ridley and Baker 1995). The sheep to which Pattison fed placental and fetal tissue came from a flock that had been especially bred to develop scrapie after being injected subcutaneously with scrapie-affected tissue. We know now that these sheep were likely to develop scrapie naturally anyway, and, indeed, the flock that Pattison used collapsed with an outbreak of natural scrapie shortly after this experiment (Pattison 1974). Thus, without the necessary control animals no one can be certain that those sheep fed placentas got their scrapie from that event, because it is likely that at least some of them were destined to get scrapie anyway. The fact that there was no difference in disease incidence between the goats (which are very susceptible to accidental transmission of scrapie) and the sheep (which are not so susceptible), nor between animals injected intracerebrally (which is a very efficient, if unnatural, method of transmission) and those infected orally (which is usually less efficient), suggests that disease may not have been caused by the placental material to which these animals were exposed.

There is a further flaw in the argument that maternal transmission explains the persistence of scrapie in the field. Even if this artificial feeding experiment did lead to scrapie in these sheep, it does not follow that all natural scrapie is caused in this way. The evidence that sheep regularly eat each other's placentas or that placental tissue contains high levels of the infectious agent is not very convincing. In one experiment no infectivity was found in ovary, uterus, fetuses, milk, colostrum (first-day milk), mammary gland, or saliva of affected sheep, using experimental transmission of disease to mice, the standard method of measuring levels of infectivity (bioassay) (Hadlow *et al.* 1979, 1982). In another experiment, it was reported that of the very many mice injected with material from the reproductive tract of scrapie-affected sheep, only a few became sick, but the data are given in tabular form only, without the full experimental details (Hourrigan 1990). Interestingly, there have been several reports of the development of spongiform encephalopathy in a few mice injected intracerebrally with healthy brain tissue. This could be due to some biological mechanism that we do not currently understand, or perhaps it could indicate how easy it is for the injected tissue to become contaminated in a laboratory that works with large amounts of scrapie-infected material. In either case these 'false positives' remind us that where only very limited data are available they should not be taken completely at face value. Until someone does all these experiments again, it is our view that the question of whether sheep 'in the field' ever catch scrapie from each other, or by grazing on contaminated land, will remain unanswered.

The idea that placentas contain sufficient infectivity to pose a risk to other flock members (following ingestion), or to the fetus by intrauterine contamination, or to a lamb following some event involving contamination during the admittedly messy business of birth and early suckling, has further important implications for our understanding of the pathogenesis (mechanism by which disease develops) of scrapie. In scrapie, the highest levels of infectivity are found in the brain because prion protein is produced in greatest amounts in the brain. Other organs of the body do produce a certain amount of prion protein and may therefore generate lower levels of infectivity. If the placenta in a scrapie-affected animal is sufficiently infectious to cause substantial lateral transmission by various mechanisms, either it produces infectivity of its own or it is 'contaminated' by infectivity carried there from elsewhere by the blood. There have been few attempts to detect infectivity in the blood of animals or humans affected with prion disease, and, reassuringly, these have rarely been successful. Placental tissue develops from the growing embryo and therefore belongs biologically (that is, genetically) to the offspring, not the mother. So if the placenta is producing its own infectious agent, the offspring of scrapie-affected sheep must be capable of generating infectivity twice, once in its placental tissue before it is born and possibly later on in adulthood if it develops scrapie itself, but not in infancy. Attempts to detect infectivity in the tissues of newborn animals have been uniformly negative. We do not know whether the placental tissue used in Pattison's feeding experiments belonged to a fetus that would have developed scrapie if it had survived to adulthood, since both ewe and lamb were sacrificed to provide the placental tissue.

One might have thought that, in order to establish the circumstances under which scrapie occurs and to assess whether the consumption of scrapie-affected meat could produce disease in humans, an exhaustive study of the distribution of the infectious agent in different tissues, at different ages, and at different times during the development of the disease in sheep, would have been undertaken. To be fair, such experiments are difficult to carry out. Until recently the existence of the infectious agent could only be demonstrated in transmission experiments, which took months and sometimes years to complete. When transmission studies were set up, using sheep as the recipient animals, the design of the experiment could be compromised. If sheep known to be susceptible to scrapie were used, a substantial proportion of them might be expected to develop scrapie naturally, and if sheep resistant to natural scrapie were used, then the sensitivity of the experiment was lost. So most experimental transmissions used mice as the recipient animals and, although the sensitivity of the tests was reduced a little, the use of mice had the advantage that experiments could be undertaken in the controlled conditions of a laboratory rather than in a field, and an almost unlimited number of animals could be used. Such experiments showed that many of the organs of the body contained low levels of infective agent. But according to Bill Hadlow, who did much of this work himself, 'the reported results have been fragmentary. Rather than treating them as tentative findings, they are accepted as established facts about the disease; they become part of the scrapie dogma. But sometimes they do not deserve that distinction' (Hadlow 1991). Nevertheless, these were the data used to inform the scientists' decisions as to which organs to include in the 'Specified Offals Ban' of 1989. This ban was designed to protect people from any risk from BSE-affected material, and forbade the inclusion of many internal organs from cattle in human food. As it would have taken several years to repeat these transmission experiments, it was inevitable that decisions had to be based on information available at the time, however inadequate. The internal organs of cattle with BSE have now been tested for infectivity in more detail and, fortunately, the data suggest either that the BSE agent is less widely distributed in the body than is the scrapie agent or that there were some 'false positive' results in the original scrapie transmission data. The Specified Offals Ban might, therefore, have been more extensive than was strictly necessary. But this was more luck than judgement.

Do sheep pass on scrapie to their offspring: the issue of maternal transmission

It is perhaps indicative of the inadequacy of the data on the lateral transmission of natural scrapie that almost no one believes that lateral transmission of BSE occurs either by contact between animals or by shared pasture or housing. Yet, despite equally inadequate data, belief in the maternal transmission of scrapie is so well established that until recently it remained completely unchallenged. How did the concept of maternal transmission become so central to the story of scrapie?

The answer lies in the fact that the probability that a sheep will develop scrapie is undoubtedly influenced by whether its mother also developed scrapie. But many sheep with scrapie do not have a mother with scrapie (although their siblings and other sheep within the flock are more likely to have scrapie than sheep from some other flock). This could all be explained if it were supposed that sheep could 'carry' scrapie infection for all of their lives without showing signs of illness, and that they could pass it to other animals, or, in other words, if a certain amount of lateral transmission occurred within flocks between sheep which were not necessarily siblings. In order to show that transmission of disease is occurring by some mechanism peculiar to the maternal relationship (for example, transplacentally, or via milk, or the close physical contact of ewe and lamb), one needs to prove that the incidence of scrapie in the offspring of subsequently affected mothers is higher than the incidence in the offspring of subsequently affected fathers. The alternative hypothesis is that the parents are passing on a genetic susceptibility to disease, in which case the incidence in the offspring of subsequently affected fathers and mothers would be the same, because the ram contributes the same amount of genetic material as the ewe. In considering the data one must take into account what actually happens in commercial flocks of sheep. It is relatively easy to identify ewe and offspring since these animals will often associate within the flock, and, in managing a flock of ewes, the sheep farmer is likely to keep records of the productivity of his ewes. But the ram may be bought in, borrowed, or sold on, and will be used to serve a very large number of ewes in one flock. It is, therefore, much more difficult to collect data on the offspring of a large number of rams. In a classic paper, the bedrock on which belief in maternal transmission rests, Alan Dickinson and colleagues (1965) reported on the incidence of scrapie in the *parents* of a large number of lambs with or without scrapie. However, on reading their report we found that only two rams with scrapie were involved in the analysis, so that the influence of scrapie in rams cannot be said to have been properly assessed. A more rigorous study was undertaken by Parry (1983) who found that almost all sheep, both of whose parents later had scrapie, themselves developed scrapie, and that those sheep, neither of whose parents nor any other known relatives later had scrapie, themselves never got scrapie. He also found that about half of the sheep, only one of whose parents had relatives with scrapie, went on to develop scrapie, *irrespective of whether that 'suspect' parent was the mother or the father*. This pattern of disease can be described as 'recessive'. All animals carry two copies (strictly speaking, *alleles*) of every gene, one inherited from the mother and one from the father. In a recessive disease, when both copies of the gene involved carry susceptibility, disease is almost inevitable. When only one copy of the susceptibility gene is inherited together with a non-susceptibility gene from the other parent, the gene carrier is likely not to be sick. But if it mates with another susceptibility gene carrier, its offspring stand a high chance of inheriting two copies of the susceptibility gene and, therefore, of developing disease. As we shall see in the next section, modern techniques of molecular analysis are allowing the genetic basis of scrapie to be firmly established, and it turns out that a gene that is equally likely to have been passed on by the ram as by the ewe contributes to the occurrence of scrapie in the offspring, irrespective of whether either of the parents themselves develop scrapie.

Table 2.1 Scrapie in the offspring of ewes and rams themselves at high, medium, and low risk of scrapie; values are percentage of offspring affected by 4–5 years of age (after Parry 1983)

	Ewes		
Rams	High risk	Medium risk	Low risk
High risk	86%	46%	0%
Medium risk	50%	17%	0%
Low risk	0%	0%	0%

Is scrapie all in the genes?

The techniques of molecular biology and molecular genetics have revolutionized biology. Whereas genetics was previously a largely theoretical subject in which the existence of different genes and different alternative forms of the same gene (copies or alleles) had to be inferred from the characteristics of the animal or person in which the gene existed, molecular techniques allow the gene to be found and every aspect of its make-up determined.

Molecular biological analysis of prion protein forms the basis of understanding how this peculiar protein causes disease. The use of molecular genetics has been no less important in our understanding of which animals or people develop prion disease under different circumstances. Although not yet complete, analysis of the PrP gene in sheep, together with the use of transgenic mice, in which copies of different PrP genes have been artificially inserted, will eventually resolve the original argument about whether scrapie is naturally a genetic or acquired disease. It turns out that the genetics of natural scrapie and the genetics of experimentally transmitted scrapie are intimately linked, though not identical. It also turns out that the genetics of scrapie depend on which breed of sheep one is considering and, since there are dozens of different breeds of sheep, as well as many cross-breeds, the situation rapidly becomes rather complicated.

Before the advent of these molecular techniques, veterinary scientists had made attempts, using Cheviot, Swaledale, and Herdwick breeds, to select lines of sheep that were resistant to experimental infection with scrapie. The most closely studied of these was a flock of Cheviot sheep which has been maintained outside Edinburgh for almost 40 years (Hunter *et al.* 1996). A large number of breeding ewes was injected with scrapie. Some developed scrapie but most did not. The lambs that had earlier been born to those ewes that developed scrapie were put in the 'scrapie-susceptible' flock and the lambs born to ewes that did not get scrapie were put in the 'scrapie-resistant' flock. Sheep in both these flocks were injected with scrapie and the lambs born to them were reassigned to the two flocks, depending on whether or not their injected mothers developed scrapie. All went well for 10 years, with fewer and fewer sheep in the resistant flock developing scrapie following injection and more and more sheep in the susceptible flock getting scrapie after they were injected. In 1970, 15 animals in the susceptible flock developed scrapie *spontaneously* and many more became sick in subsequent years. By the 1990s scientists in Edinburgh were able to analyse the PrP gene in sheep. They found that sheep that developed scrapie always carried two copies of a particular form (technically known as the genotype) of the PrP gene while sheep that never developed scrapie, *even after injection with scrapie agent*, carried two copies of another form of the PrP gene. Sheep which carried one copy of each form did not get sick spontaneously but became ill following injection with scrapie agent. David Westaway and his colleagues have analysed the PrP gene in Suffolk sheep in Canada and, again, found that natural scrapie was associated with one particular genotype, although it is a different genotype than that associated with scrapie in Cheviot sheep (Westaway *et al.* 1994*a*). The UK government has now embarked on a breeding programme to eliminate the susceptibility genes, starting with Swaledale sheep. Eliminating all susceptibility genes from the national flock will be a long process because each breed will have to be dealt with separately, and the situation in cross-breeds may be very complicated.

Scrapie is virtually unknown in Australia and New Zealand, a fact used as evidence in the argument that any genetic predisposition to disease must reflect susceptibility to an infectious agent which is only present in the northern hemisphere. But it raises the important question of what form of the PrP gene is carried by sheep in Australia and New Zealand, a question not fully answered. There are approximately 200 million sheep in Australia and New Zealand, of perhaps 30 or 40 different breeds, although most are merinos or Romneys. Many of the breeds found in those countries do not get scrapie even in Europe, and the small number of sheep from scrapie-prone breeds which do exist in Australia and New Zealand were subject to very stringent quarantine regulation and slaughter of suspected flocks on importation. In a recent comparison of Cheviot and Suffolk sheep from Britain, New Zealand, and Australia, virtually no Cheviot sheep with the most susceptible genotype were found from any of these countries (Hunter et al. 1997). A large proportion of the Suffolk sheep from all three countries carried the most susceptible genotype but, as far as we can see from the paper, none of these sheep had scrapie. This genotype, though usually associated with scrapie in Suffolks, is resistant to scrapie when it occurs in most breeds of sheep. It is possible that the antipodean Suffolk sheep differ genetically from European Suffolks in some way that has not yet been detected. Importation restrictions have ensured that there has been almost no interbreeding between Australian or New Zealand sheep and European sheep for 50 years.

Changing mums: the technique of embryo transfer

It is possible that scrapie occurs in animals of a particular genetic constitution, but that they still have to acquire the infectious agent from the environment, perhaps from the land that they live on, from the other sheep with which they mingle, or from their mother if she is carrying the disease. One way of testing this last possibility is by the technique of 'embryo transfer', in which very young embryos, comprising only a small ball of cells, are flushed out of the uterus of sheep and then implanted into the uterus of another sheep, where the embryo develops normally. Two such experiments have been conducted in Edinburgh (Foster et al. 1992, 1996). In most, but not all cases, the donor ewes were incubating scrapie, while in all cases the surrogate (recipient) ewes were scrapie resistant. All the lambs were reared in an environment which was as 'scrapie-free' as possible, but of the 19 lambs of the most scrapie-susceptible genotype (that is, those destined to get scrapie naturally if they had been brought up in an unprotected environment) all but three developed scrapie. They could not have acquired the disease from their surrogate mothers during the placental phase of gestation since their surrogate mothers were scrapie-free. Six of the lambs that developed scrapie came from donor ewes that did not get scrapie, so it is unlikely that the lambs caught the disease from them. If they did, they must have done so either at the embryo stage of development, which would preclude infection via the placenta, or during the birth process, or from the mother's milk. The fact that three of these lambs have survived has been used by some people to argue that this genotype merely confers susceptibility to 'catch' the agent, which, it is argued, is spread throughout the environment. However, these three lambs were brought up with the other susceptible lambs that did get scrapie, and should, therefore, have encountered the same level of environmental contamination. At present, the survival of these three sheep does not tell us where the agent is in the environment, nor does it exclude the possibility of scrapie being a wholly genetic disease, since many genetically determined diseases exhibit only partial 'penetrance', that is, some of the gene carriers are lucky enough to escape being sick. Time and more experiments will doubtless resolve these uncertainties.

A few mink, mule deer, and unanswered questions

A few other obscure spongiform encephalopathies of animals have long been recognized. The most important of these is transmissible mink encephalopathy (TME), which was studied extensively by Richard Marsh, a veterinarian working in Wisconsin (Marsh 1992). TME occurred as severe but isolated outbreaks (about 14 in 30 years, worldwide) in mink that were farmed commercially for their pelt. Caged mink would be fed on meat from whatever cheap source could be found. Such meat frequently came from local farmers, who would provide the carcasses of sick animals, which could include sheep, cows, or other animals. It might be thought that the most obvious explanation for these outbreaks of TME would be that sheep with scrapie were sometimes included in the food supply. In fact only one outbreak, in Finland, can be realistically related to scrapie, the remainder being a matter of assumption and conjecture. Attempts to transmit scrapie to mink have been remarkably unsuccessful. Mink injected intracerebrally with brain extracts from scrapie-affected Cheviot sheep and goats from Britain did not become sick, although transmission of disease following intracerebral injection of brain tissue from American Suffolk sheep with scrapie was successful. Whether this reflects a genuine difference between the 'strain of agent' (an important issue to which we shall return later) found in Cheviot and Suffolk sheep, or whether there is some other unsuspected difference between the two experiments is one example of the many unresolved details about prion disease research which make the subject so intriguing and so frustrating. Even more curious was the finding that none of the mink which were *fed* on scrapie-infected sheep tissue became ill, although all those that had scrapie-infected tissue rubbed into scratched (scarified) skin later developed spongiform encephalopathy. This suggests that it may not have been eating *per se* but self-inoculation while eating, which was the true route of transmission of disease in these outbreaks of TME.

Five of the 14 known outbreaks of TME occurred in 1961 on farms in Wisconsin which shared one supplier of foodstuff. This strongly suggests that the feed was the source of contamination. What was it contaminated with? One outbreak (in 1985) occurred in Stetsonville, Wisconsin, on a mink farm where, it was said, no animals had been fed sheep meat. Instead, the farmer used mainly the locally available carcasses of horses and 'downer' cows. These are dairy cows that had 'collapsed' but for which no veterinary diagnosis had been sought. Could some of these cows have had BSE? BSE has not been reported in any American cattle despite strenuous efforts at detection, and certainly does not occur in epidemic form as it does in Britain. But could BSE occur as an extremely rare, sporadic, disease of elderly cattle in much the same way as CJD occurs sporadically in the human population? BSE has been transmitted to mink both orally and by intracerebral injection of infected cattle brain, although the resulting spongiform encephalopathy seen in the mink does not look entirely similar to that seen in 'natural' TME, so this experiment casts little light on the cause of TME.

If TME is poorly understood, then another form of spongiform encephalopathy known as 'chronic wasting disease of captive mule deer and Rocky Mountain elk' is downright mysterious (Williams and Young 1980, 1982). This disease occurs in Colorado and Wyoming, and has been seen mainly in four wildlife parks which have exchanged animals. That two wholly distinct species in the same parks have been affected strongly suggests that some contamination has occurred, rather than that inbreeding has brought out a genetic disease. The source of the contamination is unknown. The disease occurs in animals reared by their mother, and in those which were hand reared on cow's milk. Apart from this milk, the animals are not known to have been fed on any animal-derived protein. Some animals grazed on grass, but others were kept in pens and were fed on rations of hay and other vegetation. The disease has also been seen in wild mule deer and elk ranging within a few square kilometres of the parks. Perhaps these animals had broken into the wildlife parks and were exposed to the same contamination. Who knows?

Can scrapie cause disease in humans? Despite the near hysterical fear of BSE which gripped some people before there was any evidence that it might be a risk to humans, little concern has ever been expressed over scrapie. This is probably because BSE is perceived as new and therefore 'unreliable' whereas scrapie is an old disease which, apparently, has caused no harm to humans in the past. Worldwide epidemiological studies have revealed no relationship between the number of cases of CJD and the number of sheep, or the incidence of scrapie, in different countries. Extensive investigations have failed to reveal any links between individual cases of CJD and the consumption of sheep products, or occupation in any part of the sheep industry, although the possibility that scrapie has occasionally caused a CJD-like illness in humans cannot be excluded. Even if BSE came from sheep scrapie in the first place, it may be a risk to humans (although this is not yet formally proven) because the transmissible agent may have changed some of its properties, including its host range, when it moved into cattle. However, experimental transmission studies using monkeys suggest that the BSE agent may be no more pathogenic in monkeys than is the scrapie agent (Baker *et al.* 1993). Alternatively, it is possible that, while the agents of scrapie and BSE are both potentially risky, we do not expose ourselves to the scrapie agent in the same way as we did to the BSE agent. Most sheep meat is eaten as 'lamb', that is, when the animal may have been too young to have had detectable levels of infectivity in its tissues, whereas various 'beef-containing' products were (until April 1996) made from the carcasses of dairy cows which were past their peak productivity. Sheep head, including the brain, which is the most infectious part of the affected animal, is a low-value product which was used mainly in the manufacture of animal feed (where it is thought to have been responsible for starting the BSE epidemic), rather than being used for human food.

In the 1970s scrapie was shown to be experimentally transmissible to monkeys by the intracerebral injection of homogenized brain tissue from affected sheep. Surprisingly, transmission to chimpanzees was unsuccessful (Gajdusek 1990). Chimpanzees, gorillas, orang utans, and humans are great apes. Apes and monkeys are collectively known as primates. It has been suggested on a number of occasions that attempts should be made to see whether BSE will transmit to chimpanzees, although the current ethical objection to using this endangered and sentient animal for such purposes has overridden the suggestion. Since the occurrence in Britain of a few cases of CJD that may be related to BSE, renewed calls have been made for this experiment to be performed. But there have been many objections from those who feel that chimpanzees are too similar to humans to be used in this way, and from those who argue that chimpanzees are not humans, and that laboratory experiments cannot model what may have happened to produce BSE-related CJD in humans.

Conclusion

The desire to understand the mode of transmission of natural scrapie nags at the heart of anyone who works on this disease. It is our view that the pattern of occurrence of scrapie within flocks, across breeds, and in different countries can be explained by the genetic make-up of the sheep in question. Whether sheep of the appropriate genotype always get scrapie spontaneously is not clear, but our understanding of the epidemiology of prion disease in humans and in 'transgenic' rodents, whose PrP genes have been artificially altered, strongly suggests that the disease can occur without exposure to an infectious agent. Transmission is easily demonstrable experimentally, and the genetics of susceptibility to infection is closely related to the genetics of spontaneously occurring disease. It is possible that some sheep have caught scrapie from each other or from heavily contaminated surroundings, although we are unconvinced by most reports that this has actually happened. We find no evidence at all for the occurrence of maternal transmission, and we are as puzzled over where the idea came from, as we are over why it will not go away. If scrapie was the source of the infectious agent of BSE, it must be supposed that the cattle population will never be safe from the return of BSE so long as scrapie remains an endemic disease in this country. The British government is now thinking seriously of ways of eradicating scrapie. There is also another reason for needing to get rid of scrapie. If scrapie can cause disease in cattle, BSE might cause disease in sheep. Such a disease might be indistinguishable from scrapie but might pose the same risk to humans as BSE. If this occurred, the British sheep industry would suffer the same fate as the beef industry. Although BSE has been experimentally transmitted to sheep under laboratory conditions, there is no evidence that BSE has passed to sheep in the national flock, but the possibility does need to be thought about urgently.

Much has happened in our understanding of scrapie in recent years, but research into the disease still has much the same 'flavour' as it had almost 40 years ago. In 1960, Tony Palmer, a respected veterinary neurologist in Cambridge, wrote a prophetic paragraph about the way in which scrapie might come to be understood (Palmer 1960). The italics in parenthesis are ours.

Evidence for the experimental transmission of scrapie to normal animals can no longer be disputed, but it would be unwise to ignore the possibility of a congenital factor that leads to a predisposition for contracting the disease. Determination of the nature of the transmissible agent is severely handicapped because laboratory animals are not susceptible. [*It is now known that they can be.*] Perhaps the use of tissue culture techniques may be profitable. [*They now are.*] But what could be the nature of this agent, an agent that can resist so many biological insults? That it consists entirely of protein is unlikely in view of its stability to heat and formalin. [*The amyloid nature of prion protein may afford such protection.*] There may be a non-protein moiety, perhaps carbohydrate [*the prion protein has certain important carbohydrate attachments*], which on introduction into the body forms a template for the subsequent reduplication of the agent. [*This is the crux of the modern theory of prion disease.*] But theories such as this must be put to the test and with scrapie this entails many months of tedious trials. If the nature of the agent causing scrapie can be finally determined the results may lead to spectacular changes in the present-day concept of the genesis of disease.

3

Kuru, a story of cannibalism

A garden of Eden

Picture, then, a garden of Eden, a tropical paradise, but one with a dark secret. The island of New Guinea has a prolific array of plants, particularly hibiscus and orchids, large colourful butterflies, and the fantastic 'birds of paradise', which have become so well-known worldwide. It is no accident that this island should have produced birds with startling plumage, whose elaborate mating displays produce splashes of colour amongst the trees. In cold and difficult climates, with animals competing for limited food and shelter, the most urgent evolutionary pressure on any animal is to survive to adulthood in order to produce offspring. But in an environment where food and shelter are plentiful, evolution progresses by sexual selection—what matters most is whether you can persuade a potential mate to choose you! It is by this mechanism that the birds of paradise have become increasingly diverse and extravagant in their courtship display.

Like many islands separated by some distance from the nearest mainland, New Guinea does not boast a wide variety of animals, and, apart from wild boar and pigs, the few animals there are have not been of great use as food for the human inhabitants. The land is mountainous, and the combination of steep terrain and dense tropical vegetation meant that valleys, which may be but a few miles apart, were effectively cut off from each other for centuries. This led to the development of hundreds of completely different languages and many isolated groups of people in the highlands who were culturally separate for many generations. It also led to another, darker aspect of this garden paradise. Where groups of people have territories which adjoin those of 'strangers', tribal warfare and blood feuds are likely to flourish. Isolated groups of people may develop customs and beliefs which vary greatly from those of other groups, and their development may not benefit from the advantages of contact with other cultures.

The 'discovery' of New Guinea

New Guinea was 'discovered' in the sixteenth century by Portuguese navigators, but it was never popular as a place for colonization because of its particularly humid atmosphere, which encouraged diseases such as malaria, especially in the lowlands, and its many different and frequently hostile, indigenous peoples. In the nineteenth century the western half of the island (now called Irian Jaya and part of modern Indonesia) was claimed by the Dutch. The south-eastern part was claimed by the British East India Company, and the north-eastern part by Germany. These eastern parts later amalgamated to form Papua New Guinea, which was administered by Australia until it became an independent Commonwealth country in 1975. During the early part of the twentieth century the lowland coastal area of Papua New Guinea was home to a few missionaries, and to a small number of settlers growing cash crops such as coffee. The more remote highland regions remained largely untouched by Western influence.

There was a further period of development after the Second World War,

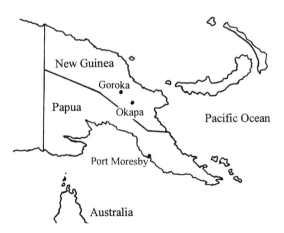

Fig. 3.1 Map of the eastern end of the island of New Guinea. The island is situated in the South Pacific, off the nothernmost tip of Australia. The western half of the island is Irian Jaya, a province of Indonesia. The capital of Papua New Guinea is Port Moresby. Kuru occurred mainly in the eastern highlands and was investigated from medical centres in Goroka and Okapa.

during which Australian administrative and medical outposts were established in the more inaccessible regions. One of these was at Okapa, and it was here, in the early 1950s, that a young German doctor, Vincent Zigas, first encountered people with a peculiar movement disorder (these are referred to as motor disorders by neurologists) that would not respond to any treatment, and which was to attract the attention of researchers from all over the world. By the end of that decade many of the key players in the story of kuru had visited Okapa. These included Carleton Gajdusek, an indefatigable American paediatrician and virologist who had been working in Australia and then in Port Moresby, the capital of Papua New Guinea, but who had found his own way into the highlands, having heard that something interesting was happening. There was also Michael Alpers, an Australian neurologist and stoical figure who, by his own admission, had found medical school 'the most stultifying experience of his life' (Alpers 1992), and who was to develop the medical service in that region and become Director of the Papua New Guinea Institute of Medical Research in Goroka. Robert and Shirley Glasse, anthropologists determined to understand the pattern of occurrence of kuru, were also important contributors.

The story of kuru has been documented in many scientific papers in the medical and anthropological literature, and a good account can be found in the many papers by Michael Alpers. The anthropologists and medical doctors cared for all of the hundreds of people with kuru who came to Okapa, or whom they visited in their home villages. They also carried out extensive investigations of the patients' histories, clinical features, and lifestyles, to build up an epidemiological picture of kuru. The disease occurred mainly in women, and in children of either sex, but was much less common among adult men. Blood relatives were frequently affected, and sometimes people who had married into an affected group also became sick. Conversely, individuals originating from an affected group often became sick at the same time as each other, even though some of them may have moved away to join another group, perhaps to get married or for some other reason. The fact that so many victims of the disease were related to each other suggested that there could be a genetic (heritable) component to the disease. However, there are no genetic mechanisms that result in disease occurring mainly in adult women, and in youngsters of either sex. Similarly, it was difficult to find a genetic explanation for the occurrence of disease in people who were related only by marriage. It was difficult to explain on the basis of exposure to an environmental agent, such as a toxin in the food, the water, or on the land, why it was that people who had moved away from an affected group many years before went on to become ill.

The origin of kuru

The origin of kuru was researched extensively by the anthropologists Robert and Shirley Glasse and others (Glasse 1967), who gathered information from 'the people who had always been old'. Since the Foré people had no written language or records, it was difficult to establish just how old someone actually was. In the early 1960s life expectancy was short and the menopause was a rare condition. It could be estimated that the majority of 'old' people were little over 40 years of age, but there were a very few people still living who were regarded as having been 'old' even when the currently old had been children. Thus, these very old people may have reached their 'three score years and ten', that is, they may have been more than 70 years old.

The first case of kuru seems to have occurred sometime in the 1920s in a village called Uwami in the Keiagana region of eastern highlands of Papua New Guinea. It was recognized as being something completely new and was regarded with some concern because it appeared to be a particularly powerful piece of witchcraft. The next case occurred a few years later in the neighbouring village of Awande, followed shortly afterwards by more cases in adjacent villages in the valley of the Lamari River. By the time of the Second World War, kuru had appeared in a large number of villages throughout the area inhabited mainly by the Foré linguistic groups. The timing of this can be established with some precision because the villagers recounted the simultaneous (but coincidental) spread of kuru and the first sightings of aircraft taking part in the Pacific theatre of war. Some aircraft crashed, and pieces of metal and other gadgets appeared among the possessions of the tribesmen. Some ammunition must also have landed, and stories of explosions were incorporated in the folk history. These events were accompanied by a major epidemic of dysentery which, unlike most of the intestinal infections that affected these people, was fatal to a large proportion of the population. It would appear, therefore, that the first contact these highland people had with 'civilization' occurred because of a war of which they knew nothing, and that our first gifts to them were guns and germs. After the war, government patrols came to the edge of the kuru region and a mission station was set up in the village where kuru had first appeared. The first written report of kuru was made in 1953 by a patrol officer, Mr J. R. McArthur (McArthur 1953).

The Foré people had by this time gained something of a notorious reputation, even though they had been rather less antagonistic to Westerners than some more remote groups. They were widely regarded as cannibals and enjoyed a reputation among other tribes and certain Westerners for possessing a particularly powerful witchcraft since they could just 'wish a person dead'. However, this undeserved reputation may have derived from the fact that, because they had had more contact with Westerners, more was known about the Foré people than about other isolated groups.

Sorcery?

The local people had their own explanation of kuru. It was assumed that, like many other illnesses and misfortunes, kuru resulted from witchcraft. The mental symptoms of the disease were perhaps particularly compatible with the idea that the victim was possessed by evil spirits. Sufferers were seen to tremble, supposedly with fear, to grimace and sometimes to collapse in helpless laughter, as if in communication with ghosts. A sorcerer, most likely a man, who was thought to have cast the spell was usually identified and frequently killed. But this ultimate revenge, or 'tukabu' in the Foré language, did not result in the recovery of the patient. At the height of the epidemic, probably in the early 1960s, kuru was the leading cause of death in women, producing a distortion of the sex ratio in favour of three men to every woman. This produced difficulties in a social system in which polygamy had been practised as a way of coping with the loss of young men in tribal warfare or by reprisal killings in response to all manner of misfortunes. Consequently, the marriage age for girls became lower and lower, many men had had several successive wives, and there were innumerable kuru orphans to be cared for.

Cannibalism?

It was widely believed by resident Westerners that the Foré-speaking people, amongst whom most of the cases of kuru occurred, had been cannibals; this view was shared by the indigenous population of Papua New Guinea. Like Michael Alpers, Carleton Gajdusek, and most others who work in the field, we see no reason to doubt that cannibalism was a feature of this culture, despite arguments to the contrary by one or two anthropologists. Cannibalism ceased fairly abruptly at the end of the 1950s, when Australian administrators set up outpost stations with patrol officers in the interior highlands. At first, cannibalism, strange or even abhorrent though it may have seemed to Westerners, was not considered to be responsible for the disease, for the simple reason that the practice was not confined to the area most affected by kuru. The type of cannibalism practised in Papua New Guinea was mainly endocannibalism, that is, the consumption of one's own relatives, particularly parents, as an act of respect and appreciation. Cannibalism was most prevalent among the northern Foré people, who claimed to have acquired the habit from their more northerly neighbours, and to have practised the endocannibalism of relatives and, occasionally, exocannibalism, that is, the consumption of people from other ethnic groups. Cannibalism seems to have appeared within the culture of the southern Foré people about 10 years before the first appearance of kuru. The bodies of those who died of 'corrupting' diseases, such as leprosy or dysentery (both of which were regarded as contagious), were not eaten, unlike the victims of kuru, who were frequently eaten because they were often young and greatly mourned, and because no ill effect came of it in the short term. Following dismemberment, the body was cooked in a variety of ways and, apart from the bitter-tasting gall bladder, all of it was eaten. The women and children ate most of the internal organs, including the brain, whereas the men, who were much less involved in the preparation of the meal, ate mainly the meat (muscle). This pattern of behaviour was compatible with the idea that kuru was associated with cannibalism, particularly of the non-muscle parts of the body, because the disease occurred mainly in women and children. But two further aspects of the epidemiology of the disease had to be considered before the relationship between cannibalism and kuru began to make sense. The first was that the time between a presumed cannibalistic event and the onset of the disease could vary from 3 years (judging by the age of the youngest victims) to more than 20 years (judging by the occurrence of kuru in adults who had moved many years before to a tribal group not otherwise affected with kuru). As time went by, the extent of the relationship between cannibalism and kuru became clearer because very few children born after the cessation of cannibalism at the end of the 1950s have developed kuru and, with each passing year, the age of new victims claimed by kuru has been increasing. A few newly diagnosed cases of kuru do still occur in the 1990s among older people in the highlands of Papua New Guinea, and this appears to suggest that, if these cases are caused by contamination during cannibalism, the incubation period for this disease can be as long as 40 years. The second aspect was the important realization that the disease was caused by an 'infectious agent' and that the epidemic had started with one infected person, that is, that every case was related by contamination to every other case, rather than to cannibalism in general.

Some people found difficulty in accepting this account of the epidemiology of kuru, not only because the disease was unknown outside the Foré region although cannibalism was not, but because cannibalism, while it might provide an explanation for the spread of disease within a group, could not explain where kuru had come from in the first place. Indeed it does not. To understand this one must remember that, in addition to being transmissible under certain circumstances, prion disease can also occur spontaneously. But even the idea that kuru might have started from a sporadic case of CJD, as is accepted by many, is worthy of some thought.

The present population of Papua New Guinea is about 4 million, life expectancy at birth is about 57 years, and 40 per cent of the population is less than 15 years of age. In the early part of this century, the indigenous, highland population would have been very much smaller and life expectancy much shorter. Since the annual incidence of sporadic CJD is only one case per million in a long-lived population, and since almost all cases are over 40 years of age, the chances of CJD occurring at all in this group of people was unlikely but not impossible. L. B. Steadman, an anthropologist who denies that kuru was maintained by cannibalism, comments that kuru was thought to have started in the early part of this century when the first Western settlers took up residence in Papua New Guinea. 'What's probably happened is that kuru is a variant of Creutzfeldt–Jakob disease, another slow virus disease, which was almost certainly introduced by the Europeans. Rather than a savage disease transmitted savagely, kuru is a European disease' (Kolata 1986). Steadman fails to grasp that CJD is not a contagious disease found only in the West, and passed between individuals by the casual contact of cuddling each other or by sharing cutlery. Furthermore, the disease is so rare as to make the probability of it occurring in the handful of European settlers who visited Papua New Guinea in the early part of the twentieth century most unlikely. He could also not cope with the notion that CJD can occur sporadically in anyone, albeit with an extremely low probability, and that such a person does not have to have acquired the disease from an 'outside' source. In one sense, however, Steadman is right. The extensive handling and dismemberment of the bodies, which the Foré women undoubtedly undertook in the company of their children, would probably be adequate to transmit the disease via scratches or sores in the skin, or via the surface of the eyes. So whether human flesh was actually ingested may not be too relevant to establishing the source of the epidemic.

It is possible that the entire kuru epidemic arose from serial contamination from one original case of sporadic CJD, although, on probabilistic grounds, this person is likely to have been a member of the indigenous population and, indeed, CJD has been reported in Papua New Guinea (Hornabrook and Wagner 1975). It is also possible that brain tissue from people who are not destined to show symptoms for many years can contain infectious levels of agent, and that cannibalism in one form or another can lead to this infection being passed on and increasing in quantity (technically, 'titre') until disease appears. Issues such as these have been discussed extensively in the wake of BSE. It is perhaps a lesson worth learning that the pursuit of an apparently wholly 'academic' subject, such as social anthropology, can sometimes be of profound economic importance in a very different arena.

Three feasts and a funeral

In an attempt to plot the occurrence of kuru and to record the fading memories of funeral practices in the 1940s and 1950s, Klitzman, Alpers, and Gajdusek set out to track down all the cases of kuru that occurred in a restricted area between 1977 and 1981 (Klitzman *et al.* 1984). They visited almost all villages in which kuru had been seen during that period, and detailed genealogies of all the cases were recorded. The older people were questioned closely as to what took place at every funeral feast that they could remember. Where more than two recent kuru victims were found, additional investigations were made to establish whether any of their relatives had died of kuru some years previously and, if so, whether the bodies had been eaten. Other people who would have been at those funerals were then identified from genealogies and these people were traced to see whether they had also succumbed to kuru. Family trees were compiled from 65 recent cases of kuru, and three important feasts in the late 1950s were identified. In the account of their investigations, published in 1984, Klitzman and his colleagues state:

In early kuru work in the late 1950s, no adult denied cannibalism, all readily discussing and describing their participation in this ritual display of love and respect for their dead relatives. Cases of cannibalism have been witnessed by government officials, missionaries, and 1 of us (D.C.G) and many court records and government patrol reports consistently document that the Foré practised this ritual. Evidence of the feasts, consisting of dismembered bodies and human bones stripped of their meat, have been observed and displayed publicly, both by the villagers themselves and in government courts throughout New Guinea. However, the most telling evidence of the practices carried out during these feasts remains the eyewitness accounts of the many Foré people who were present at them. In the current investigation, most older men and women readily spoke about the custom and reported their own participation in such events as they remembered it, without embarrassment, often with pride and as a matter of course, illuminating their respect for their dead kinsmen. However, many middle-aged informants who were still children or adolescents when the custom died out, often admitted that neighbouring villages had held such feasts but denied that their own village had. Such disavowal of any involvement has appeared in the area during the 1960s with increasing contact with Westerners who had tried to eliminate cannibalism. This contact and the prosecution of offenders against the government interdiction of cannibalism in the courts have led the Foré to assume that all Westerners view the practice and perhaps the practitioners as ignominious.

What are we to make of such a statement by three respected field workers? They have taken care to point out that only one of them claims to have personally witnessed cannibalism. Court cases the world over are emotionally charged affairs with much depending on the verdict. Accusation is met by counter-accusation, and defamation of witnesses and fabrication of evidence are all common. Elders of the group may have felt that the respect normally accorded to people of their age was slipping away in the advance of 'Western' development, and they may have been eager to depict themselves as special, and as keepers of the great traditions of their tribe by exaggerating the differences between themselves and 'youth of today'. The suggestion that younger members of the group were only willing to associate cannibalism with those from other villages does sound very reminiscent of the complaints of the more sceptical anthropologists that cannibalism was always described as occurring 'over there'. Younger people may have been keen to be seen as 'modern', and may have been more apprehensive of admitting to a practice which was actually illegal. The collection of data on a banned tribal practice was likely to be as unreliable as the collection of data on illegal drug use, illicit sex, tax evasion, or the 'black economy' in the West.

Notwithstanding these doubts, many different informants about the same funeral would explain that the body was '*katim na kukim na kaikai*' (cut up and cooked and eaten), while at another funeral the body was '*putim long matmat*' (put in grave). There was a chronological transition from the former to the latter throughout the 1950s. At the height of the epidemic in the early 1960s, kuru was the major cause of death in the Foré region, so many people would have been present at the funeral of more than one kuru victim. None the less, three clusters of cases of kuru could be traced back to three episodes in different villages, and we are indebted to the paper by Klitzman and colleagues (Klitzman *et al.* 1984) for their accounts of these episodes. (The names of the people have been abbreviated, but their kinships, ages, and causes of death are described in detail.) The first cluster was identified by the deaths, in 1976 and 1977, of two brothers, Ob and Kasis, from the northern Foré village of Awandi. As children, in 1948, they had been taken to the funeral of their aunt, Nonon, who had died of kuru. Nonon had previously moved from Awandi to Kume some miles away. Although some of her relatives in Awandi chose to go to the funeral at Kume, many did not, because the journey required them to walk near the villages of Miarasa and Yagusa with which the Awandians had a blood feud. Of 16 people from Awandi who could be traced to Nonon's funeral, 12 died of kuru, five before 1955 (when documentation of births and deaths began) and the remainder between 1957 and 1977. Thus, if these 12 people contracted kuru as a result of Nonon's funerary rites, the incubation times would have been from a few years to nearly 30 years. It is difficult to be certain of the shortest incubation periods because those adults who died shortly after this feast may have been infected at a previous funeral for which there was no living memory. However, death from kuru did occur in children as young as 4 years, suggesting that incubations of only 2–3 years were possible.

Sometime in 1953 or 1954, Ob and Kasis also attended the funeral of a more distant relative called Nen, who had died of kuru, this time in Tasongagori, a hamlet associated with Awandi. Nen's husband, Kaw, was a village leader, and the funeral was a large affair. Of Nen's 16 closest relatives, 15 were in Awandi at the time and 14 took part in the funeral. Most of these had also been at Nonon's funeral. The one person in that kinship who did not take an active part in either funeral was Kasin. Although present at the second funeral, Kasin was Kaw's second wife and tradition forbade one wife to eat the remains of another of her husband's wives. Her absence from the first feast is not explained, although she was a young woman at the time of Nen's funeral and may have married into this kinship between the first and the second funeral. Only three people who attended this funeral did not eventually succumb to kuru: Lok, who died of some other disease shortly after the funeral; Kaw's second wife, Kasin, who had only watched the funeral; and Omb, who, so the account goes, only ate Nen's hand. Although the evidence is anecdotal, it is consistent with what we know about other prion diseases. While the brain, spinal cord, and certain internal organs usually carry the infectious agent, muscle and bone do not.

A second, very large cluster of cannibalistic events was traced to Ketabi village in 1950. The funeral was held for Tom, who had originally come from the village of Ai and who had recently died of kuru. Of the 60 or more people from both villages who were present at the funeral, at least 53 eventually died of kuru, although most of these people had also attended other kuru feasts over the previous few years. Of these cases, two people stand out. Pig, who was Tom's daughter, denied ever participating in any further cannibalistic feasts, and Iy, who was only 1 year old at the time of the feast. Both developed kuru in 1978, 28 years after this feast. A further dozen or so cases of kuru occurred in these two villages between 1950 and 1980, but they could not have become affected at this feast. Either they were known to be somewhere else at the time of the feast or they were born after 1950. It is believed that there were probably no further cannibalistic feasts in Ketabi and Ai.

The third episode recounted by Klitzman and colleagues concerns two cousins, Mab and Pet, who died of kuru in 1979. Both had been to the funerals of their aunts, Ton and An, who had died of kuru in 1953 and 1954 in the village of Waisa. An had herself been at the feast of Ton, but developed kuru so shortly afterwards that she had probably acquired the disease some years earlier from another relative. At about the time of these funerals, a government policeman had been stationed in Waisa and he had put pressure on the villagers to abandon their cannibalistic practices. So the next kuru victim in the village, Kandab, was buried, but rumours persisted that some of the older women had exhumed the body and eaten it in order to carry out the appropriate rituals. The truth of this story is difficult to establish but it would seem likely that there were very few further acts of cannibalism in this village after 1954. Ten deaths from kuru occurred over the next 25 years amongst the relatives who attended Ton's and An's funerals, although two toddlers, Kase and Imen, seem to have survived.

Two people

Richard Hornabrook, one of the early directors of the Papua New Guinea Institute of Medical Research, collected detailed case notes on 434 people who died of kuru (Hornabrook 1979). We will look briefly at two of the people whose lives he knew.

The first was a woman of about 40 years of age who was brought to the clinic by the village head man about 6 months after she had begun to be rather unsteady in walking. She did not want to be examined by the doctor.

Both she and her husband had already decided that she had developed kuru as a result of the sorcery practised by someone in a neighbouring village. They thought that, if the other villagers knew about her illness, it would be more difficult to identify the culprit. Only if that person could be found was there any hope that the curse could be lifted. Observation of the patient indicated that her gait was abnormal, with steps of varying length and a tendency to place the feet too wide apart in order to maintain balance. Four months later she was quite unable to walk. She was confined to her house and was very depressed. Her speech was slurred, and her efforts to move resulted in many inappropriate movements, so that she flayed about uncontrollably. When she closed her eyes she developed an involuntary grin. A few months later she was unable to sit up, could only communicate by moving her eyes, and had difficulty in swallowing the food that she was given. At this point the doctors realized that she was in the final stages of pregnancy. She also had a severe respiratory disease which was probably tuberculosis. After a long discussion between the doctor, her husband, and other relatives, she was removed from the house and taken to Okapa Hospital where the baby was delivered by Caesarean section. Mother and baby returned immediately to their village. The woman died about 2 weeks later. The baby survived and was brought up by relatives.

Another of Hornabrook's cases was a young man, an assistant and interpreter for the Kuru Research Team. He began to notice that he became rather clumsy when he was very tired at the end of long trips to see patients. Eight months later he told the research team of his worry, and some months later it was obvious that he too was developing kuru. He became depressed and resentful, complaining that he had been picked on because he worked for the Kuru Research Team. His movements became increasingly uncoordinated, such that he could only walk with the aid of a stick. Sometimes his muscles went into involuntary spasms. Six weeks later he was found lying in his house. He was very depressed and said that, since he was going to die, it had better be quick. His speech became slurred and he seemed to be losing his memory for recent events. He resisted attempts to be fed and lost his ability to speak or comprehend Pidgin. (This is a highly modified form of English using many circumlocutions. For example, in a visit of royalty to Papua New Guinea, Prince Charles was referred to by the official title of 'Number one piccaninny, b'long Mrs Queen'.) The boy died of inanition (lack of nourishment) and pneumonia about 2 years after he had first begun to be clumsy.

The medicalization of kuru

As patients began to make use of the Okapa clinic, kuru was seen through Western eyes as a progressive neurodegenerative disease. No one identified as definitely suffering from kuru by the medical team in Okapa ever recovered. A few patients presented with floridly hysterical symptoms, having been told that they had been cursed, but these patients usually got better after a period in the relatively protective environment of a hospital ward. (A few patients in Britain have also been seen in psychiatric clinics suffering from 'delusional mad cow disease'.) The symptoms of kuru usually lasted a few weeks or months (occasionally up to a year), and consisted of a particular type of postural instability and movement disorder known as 'cerebellar ataxia'. Patients were usually unable to walk unaided. Neuropathological examination of the brain after death revealed that the cerebellum, situated at the back of the brain, was the most severely and consistently affected area. Other parts of the brain could also be involved, reflecting the generalized cerebral dysfunction seen in the final stages of the disease. Microscopically the disease showed the hallmarks of spongiform encephalopathy, namely, neuronal cell loss, intraneuronal vacuolation, proliferation of astrocytes (the non-neuronal cells of the brain that support neural activity), and a greater or lesser extent of spongiform change of the brain substance. In addition, the brains of the majority of patients showed another feature which, since it was not present in all the brains, was initially not considered to be terribly important. This was the occurrence of small deposits of an unknown substance, termed amyloid, in the form of microscopic 'plaques' or small fibrous deposits arranged like the spokes of a wheel. The word 'amyloid' means waxy, although these deposits are not, in fact, composed of wax. Many years later the presence or absence of amyloid plaques in CJD and in some of the animal forms of prion disease was to play a crucial part in the debate about whether BSE had infected a small number of people in the United Kingdom.

In addition to caring for people with kuru, visiting distant villages to investigate reports of more cases, and building up a large database on the genealogies and ages of people with kuru, Carleton Gajdusek, Michael Alpers, and a few colleagues faced the daunting task of identifying, and possibly removing, the cause of the illness. The Foré people and other related groups who suffered from kuru differed from the surrounding ethnic groups only in their language. They differed little in their dietary and occupational habits, and cannibalism was believed to be widespread outside, as well as within, the kuru region. Women from villages where kuru had occurred, frequently married men from other villages. However, even when they moved to a kuru-free village they, themselves, were likely to die of kuru. On the other hand, women from kuru-free villages who married into kuru-affected villages usually did not get kuru, although occasionally they did, when they had been there for a long time. Since the existence of different languages implied that groups had been isolated from each other for at least several hundreds of years, it seemed likely that these linguistic groups would also differ genetically. It was supposed for some time that kuru was a genetic disease, although most people seemed to realize that this was not the whole story. The best indicator of whether a person would die of kuru was whether either of his or her parents had died of kuru. The rare occurrence of kuru in someone related by marriage to a kuru victim, and perhaps originating from a different linguistic group, made the genetic hypothesis untenable. The 'best-fit' genetic model, that the disease was dominant in women but recessive in males, was implausible. Diseases caused by genetic defects on the X chromosome may appear dominant in males (who only have one X chromosome) and recessive in females (who have two X chromosomes), but there is no mechanism whereby a disease can be dominant in women and recessive in men.

In August 1959, in the midst of this ethnological catastrophe and scientific confusion, a letter from Britain arrived in Papua New Guinea. It concerned sheep and, although there were no sheep in the thickly forested highlands of Papua New Guinea, this letter was to change the direction of kuru research. It was addressed to Carleton Gajdusek, who was in Papua New Guinea, and forwarded to him from his office at America's largest medical research establishment, the National Institutes of Health in Bethesda, Maryland. It was written by Bill Hadlow, a softly spoken veterinarian, who worked on scrapie in Montana. While visiting England, Hadlow had chanced upon a poster display of the neuropathology and clinical condition of kuru, which was being exhibited at the Wellcome Medical Museum in London. He had been greatly struck by just how similar the neuropathology and the behavioural symptoms of kuru were to those of scrapie, with which he was very familiar, and he had written a now famous letter to *Lancet* journal highlighting these similarities (Hadlow 1959). Fearing a threatened printer's strike, he had forwarded a copy of his *Lancet* letter to Gajdusek. In addition to comparing the two diseases, Hadlow's letter provided three very important implications. The first was that, if kuru was like scrapie, it might be experimentally transmissible with an incubation period that could be extremely long. Indeed, Gajdusek, having already tried some very preliminary transmission experiments, had concluded that no conventional virus was involved in the disease because the injected animals had remained well for a few weeks. Hadlow's letter implied that years, rather than weeks, of observation might be more appropriate. Secondly, since scrapie was readily transmissible to sheep and goats under laboratory conditions but, in the late 1950s, had not been transmitted to other species, it seemed likely that only a species close to man would be susceptible to experimental infection with kuru. The implication was that monkeys or apes should be used. Finally, it was known that the brain and spinal cord of scrapie-affected sheep contained far more infectious agent than the rest of the body, so it was thought appropriate to try to transmit disease to animals using brain tissue from kuru-affected people as the source of infectious agent. None of this was easy to do, especially in the highlands of Papua New Guinea. Brain and other tissues had to be collected (uncontaminated by bacteria) after death from patients with kuru, preserved in ice or glycerine, and later deep frozen. This important research material was transported by light aircraft to Port Moresby, the capital of Papua New Guinea, and then by international airline to the laboratories of the National Institutes of Health in the United States, by way of Australia.

Meanwhile an animal laboratory and housing facility had to be commissioned, and suitable monkeys and apes had to be assembled. The details of this are described by Michael Alpers (1968), and by the virologist Clarence 'Joe' Gibbs, who was Gajdusek's long-time colleague, and who oversaw the primate transmission studies in America for many years (Gibbs 1992). Restrictions on the use of animals for experimental research and on the collection of endangered species were much less severe in those days. Nevertheless, this large primate facility was an unusual institution. As a result of bureaucracy and building work, some years were to pass before the performance in 1962 of the crucial experiment of injecting brain from two kuru victims (Kigea and Enage) directly into the brains of two anaesthetized chimpanzees. Nothing happened. The chimpanzees (Daisy and George, later renamed Georgette on account of a small misunderstanding) appeared none the worse for their injections and were well for many months. During 1963, several more chimpanzees, some seven in all, and as many as 75 smaller monkeys were injected with tissue from other cases of kuru or of other neurological diseases. The first of the chimpanzees to be injected with kuru-infected tissue showed signs of apathy and became withdrawn 20 months after injection. Shortly thereafter, she developed a dull expression and a drooping lip. Then she and the second animal both began to show unequivocal signs of cerebellar ataxia. They were unsteady when walking about, as if they were drunk, and, to prevent themselves from falling over, would allow only one limb at a time to leave the ground or the perch they were holding. They developed characteristic postures such as bending down to eat directly from the floor, whereas normal chimpanzees pick their food up in their hands. A large number of eminent neurologists visited them and records were kept of their daily progress. As their condition deteriorated, they were hand fed and cared for in a way which nowadays would undoubtedly fall foul of safety regulations. Joe Gibbs says of those early experiments 'I really believe the care given was to a large degree provided out of affection that we all had developed for these very remarkable animals and their loss, even in the establishment of a remarkable scientific event, was felt by the staff' (Gibbs 1992). Michael Alpers, who was so familiar with patients with kuru, wrote 'the chimpanzees showed more apathy and visual confusion than their human counterparts, but this was hard to assess objectively; and their disorientation was by no means complete, for the most bemused-looking animal in the terminal phase would still turn her head at the whisper of her name' (Alpers 1968).

When it was clear that these animals were terminally ill, excitement began to mount in the laboratory, since it was certain that a momentous discovery had been made. Elisabeth Beck, a neuropathologist working at the Institute of Psychiatry in London, flew over to Bethesda to collect the brains from these chimpanzees. Beck, who had studied sheep scrapie with James Parry, had already reviewed the brains of more than a dozen kuru patients sent from Papua New Guinea by Carleton Gajdusek. After a few weeks of histological preparation, the microscope slides were ready for examination. What Beck saw was an extremely severe spongiform encephalopathy throughout the grey matter of the brain. This differed somewhat from the pathology seen in human kuru, where degeneration of the cerebellum and intraneuronal vacuolation were seen, but where rampant spongiform change had not been observed in the earlier cases. The two pathologies were, however, sufficiently similar to indicate that a kuru-like disease had been transmitted from the patient with kuru to the chimpanzee. The disease had taken about 20 months to develop and the symptoms had lasted for about 5 months. While the animals had had neurological peculiarities for the greater part of the time, they would not have been described as 'ill' for most of that time. In 1966, Gajdusek, Gibbs, and Alpers published a report of the transmission of kuru to chimpanzees in *Nature*, considered by many to be the world's leading scientific journal (Gajdusek *et al.* 1966). Gajdusek was awarded the 1972 Nobel prize for medicine.

Was the experiment justified? The animals were carefully nursed. Even though chimpanzees are thought to be amongst the most intelligent of animals, the evidence that they can worry about the future or compare the past with the present is limited. It is most unlikely that the animals suffered psychologically, although it is difficult to be sure. Thirty years ago the extent to which many large animal species were being threatened with extinction (more from a decrease in the size of their natural habitat than from the taking of animals into captivity) was not understood, and the more sordid aspects of animal trade were not necessarily appreciated by the final users of the animals. International agreements now govern the trade and movement of endangered species. These early experiments produced a 'mind-shift' in our understanding of neurodegeneration, and started a fertile line of enquiry that has produced major advances in neurogenetics and neuropathology, and which may have implications for other very common neurological conditions such as Alzheimer's disease. Many researchers regard these early experiments as historical events about which there is little to be gained now from ethical debate. Apart from the demonstration that CJD was also a transmissible disease, the many more transmission experiments involving chimpanzees carried out at the National Institutes of Health laboratories added little to the original experimental result. It soon became clear that prion diseases could be transmitted experimentally to small, New World monkeys, and the use of chimpanzees ceased. With experience, it was possible to diagnose the illness in the monkeys at a much earlier stage of the development of the symptoms, so that it was not necessary to keep sick animals alive. Furthermore, the original demonstration that kuru and CJD were very similar to scrapie meant that the majority of experiments that were intended to elucidate the nature of human neurodegenerative disease could be done using rodent-adapted scrapie. Many hundreds of thousands of rodents have been used in these experiments, but they have all been bred for laboratory research, so that their use does not interfere with the delicate balance of wildlife ecology, and their capacity for neurological symptomatology is much less.

The disappearance of kuru

Although Western medicine could offer no cure for kuru, the disease began to disappear shortly after serious research into its epidemiology began. The manner of its going turned out to be crucially important in understanding whence it came. In the early 1960s, by which time a fairly complete picture of more than 2000 cases of kuru had been assembled, researchers noticed that kuru in very young children, which had been a striking feature of the 'discovery' of kuru, had disappeared. Every year the age of the youngest case seemed to be slightly older. Furthermore, this change was most marked in the villages and the areas where Westerners had first made contact. Within a few years kuru-affected children under 10 years of age were found only in the most remote regions. However, kuru was not really dying out, because at the same time the number of adult men with kuru began to rise and continued to do so for several years.

The discovery that the experimental transmission of kuru to chimpanzees involved long incubation periods allowed the remaining pieces of the puzzle to be fitted into place. The cause of each case of kuru was now sought in events that might have occurred some, or even many, years earlier, rather than in the contemporary environment. The disappearance of kuru in young children suggested that those events had ceased rather abruptly with the arrival of Westerners in the late 1950s. It also indicated that infected women were not passing on the disease to their children either in the womb (via the placenta) or by breast milk, because the methods of caring for babies did not change at the end of the 1950s. The kinship relationships between cases, including the occurrence of kuru in some people who had married into a kuru-affected group, suggested that the event was a family affair rather than genetic. Comparison with what was known about sheep scrapie suggested that the brain, spinal cord, and some other internal organs were more likely to be infectious than the muscle. Custom dictated that it was the women, most of whom had young children in tow, who prepared the bodies during funeral rituals, and it is generally accepted that this involved the dismemberment of the corpse. Washing was not a cultural practice in that part of the world and, since everybody involved was likely to have sores, scabies, and minor lacerations, it is inevitable that contamination would have occurred through the skin by way of these abrasions. Indeed, prion disease has been experimentally transmitted intraocularly (through the eye), intradermally (through skin), and orally (by eating). Whether the funeral rituals then went on to include cannibalism is probably not crucial to the argument that the kuru epidemic was maintained by contamination during those rituals. Cannibalism is only of great importance to moral absolutists who feel that such a practice should be equally unacceptable in any culture. It is not as if there has ever been any suggestion that people were killed for the purpose of consumption.

The fact that men took much less part in the activities of the funeral rituals probably explains why kuru was rare in adult men when the epidemic was first encountered. Why, then, did the incidence rise in young men as the epidemic itself began to wane? According to 'the people who had always been old', kuru was relatively rare for most of the first part of the twentieth century, and we see no reason for doubting this. The number of cases must have increased rapidly, exploding into a major epidemic in the 1950s. Only women and children acquired the infection, and many became sick within a few years, accounting for the pattern of the disease in these groups. Men did not acquire the disease as adults, and those adult men alive during the peak of the epidemic in the 1950s had been children in the 1930s or before, when the possibility of contamination was much lower. After 1959, there were very few new infections because the cannibalistic practices had been forbidden by the Australian administration, but throughout the 1960s and 1970s many adult men who had acquired the infection as children in the 1950s became sick. By the mid-1980s, only a handful of new cases of kuru occurred each year, so the incidence was greatly reduced compared with that at the end of the 1950s, when some 200 of the Foré people died from kuru each year, and more than 90 per cent of all deaths in women were from kuru. One or two cases of kuru still occur each year in the Foré region and, in a recent interview on British television, Michael Alpers, who still cares for these patients as he has done for more than 30 years, said sadly that he had hoped to be around to see the last case of kuru, but that he now thought it unlikely. Those few new cases of kuru that he sees represent the tail end of a very long incubation period, so that what Gajdusek once called 'galloping senescence of the juvenile' has once again become an obscure disease of the elderly. Or has it?

Iatrogenic spongiform encephalopathy, the 'Western kuru'

It always comes as a profound shock to learn that some dreadful event has happened as a result of human error, and no more so than when illness or disease is caused by attempts to improve human health. Iatrogenesis (from the Greek for 'caused by a doctor') is now recognized as an important cause of CJD. The first report of such a case came in 1974 when it was revealed that a middle-aged woman had died from CJD after having had a corneal transplant some 2 years earlier. Corneal grafting, in which the corneas are removed from cadavers immediately after death, for subsequent use in those whose own cornea is damaged, is now a routine procedure, usually conducted with great success. In the case of this unfortunate woman, the donor was later found to have died of CJD. This case was only the first of a number of such reports. In 1977 an account was given of two young patients who developed CJD, 16 and 20 months after having electrodes lowered into their brains to identify the focus of electrical activity associated with epilepsy. It became clear that these same electrodes had been used in a surgical procedure on the brain of a patient with CJD, and it seems that, despite the use of standard protocols for sterilizing electrodes, they retained sufficient infectious agent to transmit disease to the two youngsters. In fact, researchers in Gajdusek's laboratory at the National Institutes of Health in Bethesda were able to transmit spongiform encephalopathy (SE) to chimpanzees using these same electrodes.

These cases, however, are unlikely to have been the first examples of iatrogenic CJD. Some 40 years ago, three patients died from CJD less than 2 years after having had neurosurgery at the National Hospital for Nervous Diseases in London, and it was later established that in each case the surgical instruments had been used beforehand for neurosurgical procedures on CJD patients. A similar account from France documents CJD in a patient whose illness developed some 2 years or so after surgery using instruments which were probably used to treat a patient with CJD some days earlier. It is clear from these reports that, if the infectious agent associated with CJD is introduced directly into the brain, by what is essentially an intracerebral injection, or to a near brain site, as in the case of corneal grafting, the incubation period from contamination to onset of illness is about 18 months to 2 years. With this sort of time lag it is difficult, but not impossible, to investigate causal relationships between the use of instruments in one patient and disease in another. What would happen if the time lag were very much greater?

Table 3.1 Iatrogenic Creutzfeldt–Jakob disease

Procedures associated with iatrogenic CJD
   Treatment with human pituitary-derived growth factor
   Treatment with human pituitary-derived gonadotrophin
   Corneal transplantation
   Intracranial use of electrodes for neurophysiological assessment
   Neurosurgery
   Neurosurgical use of dura mater (meningeal) tissue
Procedures not associated with iatrogenic CJD
   Blood transfusion
   Treatment with synthetic hormones in contraceptives or hormone replacement therapy
   Treatment with synthetic growth hormone
   Use of insulin from any source
   Transplantation of peripheral organs, for example, heart, liver, kidney, etc.
   Use of any other legal biomedicinal product

In the exciting post-war period of medical research (some might say the heyday), when biochemistry was in the ascendant, scientists devised a method for extracting hormones from human pituitary glands collected at post-mortem. This tiny gland sitting at the base of the brain is responsible for regulating many of our bodily processes, by releasing into the bloodstream chemical messengers, or hormones, which act on other body organs to ensure their smooth running in response to demands of one sort or another. One such hormone is human growth hormone (hGH), which controls the rate of growth in childhood. Another is gonadotrophin, which regulates sexual reproductive mechanisms. Pituitary-derived hormones such as these became major tools for the treatment of those whose pituitary glands failed or had to be removed, usually as a result of surgery for tumours in childhood. Untreated, such children would not achieve their full growth potential and would also be afflicted by other signs of poor development. Treatment normally consisted of intramuscular injections of hGH preparations once or twice a week, often for many years, until the endocrinologists judged that further benefit was unlikely. Replacement therapies like this have long been part of the medical repertoire and have had a good safety record. For example, many thousands of diabetes sufferers have kept the worst symptoms of their illness at bay by giving themselves injections, often twice daily, of insulin, usually prepared from pig tissue. Those who suffer from underactive thyroid glands know well the benefit deriving from replacing the missing hormone, thyroxine.

In 1984, a 21-year-old man in California complained of 'dizziness'. He had suffered all his life from the effects of deficiencies of thyroid hormone, insulin, and growth hormone, and had been treated with replacement hormones. It was thought at the time that he was hypoglycaemic and he was treated accordingly. This episode was just the beginning of a long deterioration in his health and a series of referrals to different doctors followed. Although he had marked cerebellar symptoms (the cerebellum is important in organizing motor co-ordination and balance), a diagnosis of possible CJD was entertained but then rejected because of his youth. After his death some short time later a full neuropathological examination of his brain confirmed that he had indeed suffered from CJD and prompted those who had cared for him to consider that his illness might have been related to his earlier 14-year history of growth hormone treatment. At about the same time a few other young people who had received growth hormone injections some time earlier in their lives were developing cerebellar dysfunction and were dying, although without the gross dementia seen in classic CJD. Although CJD was not considered in these cases, it was confirmed post-mortem. By now the authorities responsible for the use of pituitary-derived growth hormone in the United States had been alerted to the possibility that this treatment might be causally related to the development of CJD, and committees were set up to investigate this possibility. America was not alone in suspecting a link between CJD and growth hormone treatment. In 1985, a group of physicians in the UK reported the case of a 22-year-old woman who developed a dementing illness and marked cerebellar ataxia. Her condition deteriorated over the course of a year, by which time she had become mute and unresponsive. A clinical diagnosis of CJD was made and confirmed at autopsy. This woman had had a craniopharyngioma (a tumour associated with the base of the skull) removed at the age of 2 years, resulting in a loss of pituitary function, and between the ages of 10 and 14 she had been treated with pituitary-derived growth hormone. These cases and a number of others were described more fully in a lecture delivered by Paul Brown to the Lawson Wilkins Pediatric Endocrine Society in Anaheim, California in May 1987, in which he detailed the investigations leading up to the awful realization that CJD could be awaiting those who had been treated with growth hormone many years before. Paul Brown has been involved in research in the prion diseases for many years and remains the doyen of prion epidemiologists. A revised version of his lecture has been published and is worth reading in full (Brown 1988).

Very shortly after the early reports of a possible link between growth hormone treatment and the development of CJD were published, human pituitary-derived hGH was withdrawn from circulation and its use banned in the USA and the UK. Fortunately a suitable alternative was available since growth hormone could now be biosynthesized using the new methods of genetic engineering, and this recombinant hormone is now widely used. In the 10 years since the first cases were recognized almost 100 people have died from growth hormone-associated CJD worldwide. Unlike the 1.5–2-year incubation period in those who developed CJD after receiving direct intracerebral contamination, the incubation period in the hGH cases averaged some 12 years with a range between 5 and 30 years (calculated by Paul Brown from the mid-point of the hGH therapy). Most of these cases, like those reported earlier, presented with signs of cerebellar dysfunction, with dementia a later feature, and it has been considered that the difference between cases of sporadic CJD, which usually present with cognitive dysfunction (signs of mental deterioration), and these iatrogenic cases reflects the peripheral route of contamination in the latter. At the time it seemed surprising that a disease as rare as CJD could give rise to a sufficient number of contaminated pituitary glands to cause so many iatrogenic cases and, again, we are indebted to Paul Brown for setting the figures straight. His arguments are based on figures from the USA, with a population of some 250 million and with an annual incidence of one CJD case per million of the population. This yields a average of about 250 deaths from CJD each year in the USA. But about 1 per cent of the population dies each year, a total of 2.5 million, from which it can be seen that about 1 in 10 000 deaths each year is due to CJD. Not all deaths are accompanied by a post-mortem examination, although in the case of unusual diseases such as suspected CJD, which can be confirmed by neuropathological analysis, the probability that there will be a post-mortem is higher. Brown reports that according to surveys of some large hospital neuropathology departments the number of autopsied cases found to have CJD could be as high as 1 per 1000, and that, since 500 000 pituitary glands were processed for the extraction of growth hormone in the USA, between 25 and 250 of these could have come from CJD sufferers. Furthermore, since several thousand pituitaries were processed in each preparation, it seems likely that the contamination of the hGH was probably widespread. It now remains to be seen how many of those treated with this pituitary-derived hormone will go on to develop CJD. In the USA almost 10 000 people received this therapy, and the figure for the UK is a little under 2000. Already differences are emerging between countries where hGH has been used for many years. In the USA the proportion of hGH-treated subjects that have gone on to develop CJD stands at about 1 in 500, with a mean incubation period of 18 years, while in the UK it is about 1 in 100 with a mean incubation of 12 years, and in France it is 1 in 50 with an incubation of some 8 years. These figures suggest that the level of contamination of the hGH preparations used in France was considerably higher than in the UK and even more so than in the USA. It may be that more infected glands were used in the preparation of hGH or that the processing used was less efficient in inactivating the infectious agent, which it must be presumed was contaminating this material.

Was it never suspected that the use of growth hormone prepared from the human pituitary tissue and processed in batches of several thousand might present a risk of disease transmission? Some years before the first hGH-CJD cases appeared, researchers in Edinburgh had recognized this possibility and had carried out experiments to assess the degree of inactivation (destruction or elimination) of the transmissible agent by the processes used in the extraction of hGH, although it seems that the results of these experiments were not published until after the first hGH-CJD cases were reported. At the time of their experiments a number of different methods of hGH extraction were in use in the UK, some of which used frozen pituitary glands as the starting material, while others prepared hGH from glands that had been dried using the solvent, acetone. The latter methods required fairly harsh chemical treatments of the dried tissue and, although it produced reasonably good yields of hGH, the final product was also somewhat immunogenic, that is, on occasion it produced an adverse reaction in the patient. The former methods produced highly purified, less immunogenic hGH but, since the process was far less chemically severe, there was always the risk of infectious material surviving the extraction procedures. The Edinburgh scientists (David Taylor and his colleagues) set up experiments in which they added hGH prepared by the frozen-tissue method to a mixture of one human pituitary and some brain tissue from a scrapie-affected mouse. To ensure that the human pituitary gland donor did not have CJD they chose a patient who had died at less than 50 years of age from a brain tumour and whose neuropathological examination showed no evidence of CJD. Having homogenized the mixture, they first checked that it was infectious by injecting mice intracerebrally and then they took it through all the hGH purification steps, sampling for infectivity at each stage. By the time they had carried out all the steps in the process they were unable to detect infectivity using the mouse bioassay (experimental transmission of disease to mice), and pointed out in their report in *Lancet* that 'Our findings indicate that hGH prepared by the Lowry procedure should be safe, providing that rigorous precautions are taken to avoid laboratory contamination by the CJD agent'. It seems from their report that they believed that large-scale hGH preparations for therapeutic use had probably become contaminated during laboratory handling, possibly after the hGH had been extracted, since they went on to say 'It is likely that any hGH production laboratory where these handling problems were not understood and which had received CJD-infected pituitary tissue, would have become contaminated' (Taylor *et al.* 1985). We shall never know whether this was the case. But one thing can and should be learnt from this (and other) experiments. In bioassays, the usual measure of infectivity in a preparation is the number of animals that develop disease after being injected, and the time taken for that to happen. It is a risky business to assume that, because all of a few (or a few hundred) laboratory animals survive, it is safe to go ahead and administer the same material to perhaps many thousands of humans.

In addition to the hGH-CJD cases, there have been a few cases of CJD amongst women who have received injections of human pituitary-derived gonadotrophin for the treatment of infertility, sometimes many years earlier. However, since far fewer people have been treated with this material, it is not expected that it will be a major iatrogenic cause of CJD, distressing though it is for those who have been treated. We would point out that the vast majority of women treated with gonadotrophins and other reproductive hormones have not been given anything derived from humans and are therefore at no risk.

During 1987 another player entered the stage of iatrogenic CJD. In the *Morbidity and Mortality Weekly Report* (*MMWR*), a publication designed to notify the medical community in the USA about the adverse effects of therapy, CJD was described in a 28-year-old woman who became ill 19 months after she had had surgery to remove a cholesteatoma, a cyst-like mass within the middle-ear area. The surgical procedure had made use of a commercially available human dura mater graft during reconstruction. Dura mater (or meninges) is the tough membranous material which covers the brain. It can be stripped off at post-mortem and freeze-dried for subsequent use in a number of surgical procedures. Although it is used mainly in neurosurgical procedures, it is also used in orthopaedic surgery, orthodontics, dentistry, ear surgery, urology, gynaecology, and cardiac surgery. *MMWR* gives this list in full to alert those who have used dura mater grafts in procedures far removed from brain or head surgery to be on the look out for neurological signs in their patients. The number of cases of CJD linked to the use of dura mater has risen to about 25 worldwide, although the reader should bear in mind that such figures are likely to be out of date very quickly. Most of these cases have involved grafts in the context of head surgery and, in all but two cases, the freeze-dried dura mater had been prepared and distributed in the early 1980s by the same German company. Such is the widespread distribution of such special preparations that dura mater-CJD cases have appeared all over Europe, North America, Australasia, and the Far East, and as we write this section we have just learned (from *Lancet*, 2 November 1996) of a case in France in a 52-year-old woman who had received a dura mater graft some 11 years before developing CJD. In this case, however, there is a major complication which we will come back to in a later chapter.

4

Creutzfeldt–Jakob disease, the emergence of a clinical entity

Another disease joins the club

The brains of Daisy and Georgette, the two chimpanzees to which kuru had been transmitted, were examined microscopically by Elisabeth Beck at the Institute of Psychiatry in London, Igor Klatzo at the National Institutes of Health in Bethesda, Meta Newman at St Elizabeth's Hospital, Washington, and several other eminent neuropathologists. Igor Klatzo and Meta Newman both commented that these brains looked remarkably similar to brains that they had occasionally examined from patients with an obscure and poorly described neurodegenerative condition, sometimes called Jakob–Creutzfeldt disease. No suggestion had ever been made before that this condition might have an infectious cause. The neurodegenerative changes in these patients were more similar to those seen in other dementias of old age than to the inflammatory neuropathology seen in viral encephalitis. But the appearance of the chimpanzee brains, following transmission of kuru, was so similar to those of patients with so-called Jakob–Creutzfeldt disease that researchers in Gajdusek's laboratory immediately attempted to transmit disease from a human case of this type. (At some point this disease became universally known as Creutzfeldt–Jakob disease or CJD.) The experimental procedures followed were similar to those used in the kuru transmissions, and within 2 years the transmissibility of CJD to chimpanzees was established (Gibbs *et al.* 1968).

Creutzfeldt's first case

A little German girl, Bertha E, was only nine when her mother died of an unspecified illness in about 1900. The girl was sent to an orphanage in Breslau and at the age of 11 she became difficult, moody, and probably anorexic. By 16 years of age she was uncoordinated and her movements were jerky. Although she returned to school for brief periods, she subsequently developed delusional ideas, became disorientated, and would frequently lapse into uncontrollable laughter. She deteriorated slowly until, aged 22, she was confined to hospital for the last time and died 7 weeks later. Seven years after her death her doctor, Hans Creutzfeldt, published a report of this unusual case, which included a description of the neurodegenerative changes that he saw in her brain (Creutzfeldt 1920).

Jakob's cases

In the early 1920s, another German doctor, Alfons Jakob, compared Creutzfeldt's first case to several of his own patients (Jakob 1921). One middle-aged man and his sister died of a similar disease within a couple of years of each other. No definitive diagnosis could be made but it was clear that these people had not had a conventional viral encephalitis, and, in addition to 'Jakob's disease' or 'Creutzfeldt's disease' the term 'spastic pseudosclerosis' was sometimes used to describe their condition. In the light of contemporary views of the clinical and neuropathological appearance of the transmissible spongiform encephalopathies, the majority of these cases would clearly now be diagnosed as CJD, but some would be unlikely to satisfy modern diagnostic criteria for CJD. Indeed, in the case of Bertha E, the very young age at onset and some of her unusual symptoms, together with the rather non-specific changes reported in the brain (and the lack of those changes now regarded as specific for CJD), make it unlikely that Bertha suffered from what would now be called CJD! This is also possibly true of two of Jakob's early cases (Ironside 1996a). The unexplained early death of Bertha's mother raises the possibility of an inherited disease. On the other hand, the brother and sister, reported by Jakob, have now been shown by molecular genetic analysis to have been members of a family which suffers from an inherited form of prion disease (Brown et al. 1994).

The emergence of a disease entity

Between the 1920s and the 1960s there was a painstaking accumulation of cases which shared common features, including an age at onset usually younger than that seen for other neurodegenerative diseases and a disease progression which was usually extremely rapid. The neuropathological picture involved intraneuronal vacuolation, gliosis, neurone loss, and the development of a particular spongy appearance to the brain, which, though not unique to these cases, was highly characteristic. The term 'usually' appears in these descriptions because, apart from the invariably fatal outcome, many of the patients did not exhibit all the characteristic features, and there was considerable doubt surrounding the diagnosis. In fact, a group of British neurologists and neuropathologists questioned 'whether the syndrome is more than a convenient dumping ground for otherwise unclassifiable dementias with interesting cross relations to certain systemic degenerations?' (quoted in Kirschbaum 1968, p.14). This prompted the American neurologist, Walter Kirschbaum (1968), to publish a monograph in which he described almost all the known cases of CJD. This work is remarkable in that it identifies many of the subsequently rediscovered subtypes of prion disease, which can now be differentiated with the aid of modern methods of molecular genetics and immunohistochemistry (a process by which specific proteins can be visualized in tissues). About 10 per cent of cases were familial in the sense that at least one other close relative had died of a similar disease. This was not surprising at the time, since the transmissible nature of the disease was not known, and many other neurodegenerative diseases, for example, Alzheimer's disease, have familial and sporadic forms. It was supposed that these familial cases had been inherited.

Kirschbaum described several subtypes of CJD. These included the so-called Brownell–Oppenheimer variant, in which the early symptoms comprised a cerebellar ataxia (a difficulty in walking and maintaining balance because of damage to the cerebellum), with mental symptoms appearing only later in the disease. This variant is interesting in that it resembled kuru, the cases of CJD acquired from growth hormone (which did not appear until the 1980s), and, to some extent, the cases of 'new variant CJD' recently identified in the UK and tentatively associated with the BSE epidemic. The most rapidly progressive subtype was sometimes described as Nevin–Jones syndrome or 'subacute spongiform encephalo-pathy'. Heidenhain's syndrome was similar in that the disease course was very rapid but it had the added feature that the patient became blind, not because there was damage to the eyes but because of degeneration of the part of the brain (the primary visual cortex) that interprets the messages coming in from the eyes. One of those described as a Heidenhain case was a man whose apparently sporadic illness struck at a young age. This case was to make a dramatic reappearance nearly 40 years later when it was found that he had at least 52 affected relatives.

A further few cases were described as having neuropathology confined mainly to the thalamus (a large nucleus in the centre of the brain). This subtype, subsequently called 'fatal familial insomnia', was also destined to make an important contribution to our understanding of the genetics of prion disease. Even after all these subtypes had been identified (often by neurologists or neuropathologists seemingly eager to attach their name to a new disease), there remained a substantial proportion of cases which were still 'atypical'. Some of these would now be recognized as misdiagnoses, but others would be classified as 'atypical prion diseases', which, although they do not fulfil the other diagnostic criteria in terms of clinical presentation and neuropathology, are recognized as prion diseases because the involvement of prion protein can be demonstrated by immunohistochemical techniques. Thus, from the first descriptions by Jakob and Creutzfeldt, CJD emerged as a specific disease entity which became sharply delineated

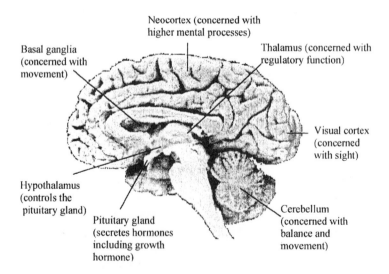

Fig. 4.1 Midline section through a human brain, showing the inner surface and indicating some of the anatomical areas mentioned in this book.

from other neurological entities because of its transmissibility. It was not, however, until 1979 that Creutzfeldt–Jakob disease appeared as an entry in the *International classification of diseases* (an official document that determines, for example, what may be put on a death certificate). It now seems, however, that the transmissible spongiform encephalopathies may be only the core of a wider group of diseases, some cases of which are neither transmissible nor spongiform, but which have in common the involvement of prion protein. It may be that in a few years time other groups of diseases will be recognized in which a variety of proteins take on a particular pathological form, and that these will join the group of prion diseases as members of a new class of disease for which a new name will be necessary.

The demonstration of the experimental transmissibility of CJD was hailed as a great breakthrough because it appeared to point towards a cause for these diseases, and experimental transmission in individual cases became extremely important in defining the limits of what came to be known as the 'human transmissible spongiform encephalopathies'. So, for a period of more than 20 years after the first demonstration of transmission of CJD, an enormous number of transmission experiments, using a limited number of chimpanzees, several hundred monkeys of various species, and thousands of animals of various other species, including many different types of rodent, were undertaken. For individual patients the demonstration of experimental transmissibility was unequivocal evidence that the disease belonged within the group containing CJD and kuru. Transmission was also attempted from many cases of other neurodegenerative conditions, including Alzheimer's and Parkinson's diseases, in an attempt to see whether they might also be caused by a transmissible agent. With one or two notable, and unreplicable, individual exceptions, which were probably due to laboratory error, no other well-recognized disease entity in humans joined the club of transmissible spongiform encephalopathies. Transmissibility became a kind of 'ring fence' which set these diseases apart from other neurological conditions. It was not until the 1980s that the involvement of prion protein became more important than experimental transmissibility in identifying the full spectrum of the disease entity.

Problems with the cause of CJD

Transmissibility did more than just 'ring-fence' this group of diseases. It imbued them with a notoriety that was to be enhanced by the arrival of BSE. To neuropathologists, the realization that for many years, and often with scant regard for safety precautions, they had been dealing with a disease that could be fatal long after it had been first encountered was disconcerting, to say the least. The occurrence in 'perfectly normal people' of a disease that was otherwise seen in cannibals was also worrying.

That the brains of people with an inherited disease contained an agent capable of experimentally transmitting disease seemed scientifically impossible. The appearance of most cases of CJD 'out of the blue' was almost as bad. Several misconceptions can be identified which led to this sense of unease. The demonstration of experimental transmissibility led to the assumption that all cases were acquired by infection, and the difficulty in establishing a link between known cases led to the view that the disease could be transmitted by the most transient social contact. Familial cases were attributed to transplacental infection or, worse still, to contamination of mother's milk. (This ignored the fact that familial cases were just as likely to have an affected father as an affected mother when allowance had been made for dubious or unknown paternity.)

Experimental transmission also led to the supposition that the disease was caused by a 'slow virus', which caused very slowly progressive damage, without the person or animal mounting the sort of immune response that is typical of an acute infection. As a hypothesis to explain transmissibility, the idea that the infectious agent was a virus was fine since, at that time, infectious diseases were known to be caused only by bacteria and viruses. It could be readily demonstrated that bacteria were not involved since these can be seen under the microscope, but exploring the possibility that a virus was involved was more difficult. Nevertheless, scientists tried to identify a virus or to find biochemical evidence of viral infection for many years, without success. This failure to find a virus led to a curious retrenchment by some scientists. It would be circular to argue that transmissibility itself proves that a virus is involved, but this has not deterred the few scientists who still maintain that CJD and the other spongiform encephalopathies are infections caused by 'slow viruses', from putting forward as their main piece of evidence the undeniable fact that these diseases are transmissible. When it became clear that the infectious agent did not behave like a conventional virus, a new concept—the unconventional virus—crept into the arena. This allowed the viral hypothesis to resist any evidence that showed that the infectious agent lacked any specific features of viruses. However, reviewing 50 years of working with scrapie, Iain Pattison (1988) pointed out that the 'use of this ingenious cover-up for uncertainty made "virus" meaningless— for is not a cottage an unconventional castle?'

The demonstration of transmissibility also led to a preoccupation with studying the transmissible agent rather than the disease itself. There were many issues to be addressed, including the relationship between amount of infectivity in tissue (measured by how much an homogenized tissue could be diluted before it no longer produced disease in animals following intracerebral injection) and the incubation period (time between injection and sickness), and the ease with which disease could be experimentally transmitted between species. This line of enquiry was somewhat problematic. When disease was transmitted from one species to another it frequently changed some of its characteristics. For example, the distribution of the pathology in the brain of the new species (host) might be different from that seen in the old species (donor). Sometimes the disease (or more correctly the transmissible agent) changed so much that it would not then transmit back to the species it had come from in the first place. The preoccupation with the infectious agent, which, as we have said, was regarded by many as an autonomous organism, led to the view that all these characteristics could be explained solely in terms of the infectious agent, and that when they appeared to change, the infectious agent must have mutated. In attempting to identify and describe the different agents from cases of CJD (kuru was remarkably well behaved in comparison), and from sheep with scrapie, a whole industry of transmissions between species and strains of mice was set up which had the effect of generating more and more data and new 'strains' of agent without establishing precisely what kind of an agent was being studied.

The worldwide occurrence of CJD

Meanwhile, Carleton Gajdusek's laboratory was drawing together its immense database of accumulated knowledge about the transmissible spongiform encephalopathies. A series of papers was produced, first by Colin Masters, an Australian neuropathologist who was visiting this laboratory, and, subsequently, mainly by Paul Brown, who was a member of Gajdusek's group for many years. The first paper attempted to explain the difference between the spongiform change seen in CJD and that seen in some other neurodegenerative diseases (Masters and Richardson 1978). This was not entirely successful, since individual cases can still be a source of diagnostic uncertainty and the detection of prion protein in brain by modern techniques has broadened the limits of the disease beyond that which was identified in those days. The second paper looked at the worldwide occurrence of CJD (Masters et al. 1979). Whereas in 1968 Kirschbaum had only been able to document 150 cases, in 1979 Masters reported on nearly 1500 cases. Some of this increase in interest was probably generated by the transmission of CJD to chimpanzees, reported in 1968. One thing was obvious from this large survey of known cases. Wherever you looked for CJD you would find it, but it was exceedingly rare. More CJD cases were found in wealthy countries, but common sense suggests that the correct diagnosis of such an unusual disease is more likely to be made in countries with an advanced medical service. In the cases documented by Masters the average age at death was 58 years. Countries which supported a good life expectancy would, therefore, have more cases than countries in which life expectancy was low. The number of cases also seemed to increase with time, but this was probably attributable to an increasing average age of the population and developing awareness of the disease amongst the medical profession. There was a slightly higher rate in urban areas than in rural areas, and the possibility was entertained that the disease was being passed from person to person by the close contact of city life. However, city dwellers are more likely to be admitted to a specialist hospital and to receive a more sophisticated diagnosis than those referred to a rural hospital (though the standard of palliative, terminal care may be the same in both cases).

There was no difference in the number of men and women that were affected and many professions were represented. The disease affected people who might have been in contact with cases of CJD, such as doctors and nurses, and others who might have been in contact with scrapie-affected sheep, such as farmers and their spouses. Among the cases there were also those, such as builders, civil servants, and sales assistants, who were unlikely to have been exposed to affected people or animals. Since it was already known that a very few cases of CJD had been acquired from contaminated instruments during surgery, considerable attention was paid to the surgical treatments that those on Masters' list had undergone. Indeed, many had undergone some sort of surgery during their life and a surprising number of these operations were neurosurgical. However, it was difficult to get control data indicating how much surgery people of a similar age and social class had also undergone, so it could not be proved that surgery was a risk factor.

The epidemiological data provided in Colin Masters' paper, and in others from different laboratories, did indicate the existence of 'clusters' of CJD, that is, two or three cases occurring within one geographical area within a few years of each other. With a disease as rare as CJD, any coincidences of this type were unlikely to have arisen by chance. This did not mean that an environmental cause for the disease had been established. CJD was found in

Australia, where scrapie was believed to have been eradicated, and in Japan, Chile, Brazil, and other countries that were not known to have scrapie. The incidence of CJD was not particularly high in Europe or Iceland, where scrapie was common. Clusters were described in Czechoslovakia, Chile, Italy, and the UK but, as we shall see later, a genetic explanation has now been found for most of these clusters. Even where it cannot be proved that cases are related, it should be remembered that in those places where the population may have increased rapidly in the previous century many people will be distantly related.

Colin Masters' next paper was concerned with familial cases of CJD and Alzheimer's disease, and those cases of CJD which occurred in families in which a large number of other members had dementing illnesses, usually diagnosed as Alzheimer's disease (Masters *et al.* 1981*a*). About 15 per cent of CJD cases were thought to come from families in which another case of CJD had also occurred. Eleven cases of familial CJD had been transmitted to monkeys, making it undeniable that the familial forms were transmissible. Apart from a slightly earlier average age at onset, the familial cases diagnosed as CJD were indistinguishable from sporadic cases of CJD. This is not too surprising because, by that time, the clinical and neuropathological description of 'definite', 'probable', and 'possible' CJD were well established, so that cases necessarily conformed to these criteria. What was less distinct was the diagnosis of illness in the relatives. To some extent this reflects the fact that the most extensive documentation was likely to be attached to the 'proband' (the case which had come to the attention of Colin Masters) and around whom the affected relatives were arranged. But this observation was also a portent of what was to come, namely that CJD belonged to a wider class of diseases, later to be called prion diseases, where the clinical symptoms and neuropathological picture were much more varied than those falling within the definition of CJD at the beginning of the 1980s. Where the family trees were large, it could be seen that the disease occurred in a 'dominant' pattern, that is, one in which about half the offspring of an affected case became sick. Where the family tree was small, this pattern could not be proved, but the data were consistent with this mode of inheritance. In some cases it was possible to identify 'obligate carriers' of the trait. These are people who, because of their position in a family tree, must have been carrying the implicated gene but for whom evidence that they had the trait is missing. For example, if a man's brother and his own child were both affected, the man must also have carried the gene. In some cases these 'obligate carriers' had died at an early age, for example, as soldiers in the Second World War, or from an accident or cancer, but in other cases they had been very old when they died of a neurological illness which, because of their age, had been described as senile dementia, or, if the disease was very rapid, as 'stroke'. These cases all suggested that there might have been a wider degree of disease presentation than was appreciated at the time. Many of the probands were first-generation American immigrants and they had died of the same illness as one of their parents, many of whom had come from eastern Europe. Affected siblings usually died at the same age rather than at the same time. In one family, two siblings were separated shortly after the birth of the younger and never met again. Forty years later they both died of CJD in the same year.

These sad stories suggest that there is little in the environment to influence the inevitable occurrence of familial CJD. There are a very few so-called 'conjugal' cases, related by marriage, that raise some doubts about this claim. Professor Brian Matthews, an Oxford neurologist who supplied the first CJD brain for transmission studies, commented on three patients who developed CJD after marrying into families in which other cases of CJD had occurred (Matthews 1985). However, in each case the person they *married* was not affected. Rather disease occurred in some other, much more distant, in-law. In each case, the patient had married a person whose family was affected with *multiple* cases of CJD. When people marry, they tend to choose people from the same geographical area and of the same social class, religious denomination, and general outlook on life, and the chances of unknowingly marrying someone who is a distant cousin is quite high. This can be measured as the 'coefficient of in-breeding' and even in places as culturally mixed as Britain it can be surprisingly high. These people could, therefore, have been carrying the same disease-associated genetic trait as the family into which they married. These cases, therefore, provide little evidence that the infectious agent of CJD can be passed between individuals who have very limited contact with each other. CJD has never been seen in anyone who was the husband or wife of a person with CJD, strongly suggesting that it cannot be passed from person to person by normal, including sexual, contact.

The puzzle of the Libyan Jews

In 586 BC, Nebuchadnezzar, the King of Babylon, captured Jerusalem and destroyed the Temple of Solomon. The Jewish people fled into Egypt, North Africa, and the deserts surrounding ancient Palestine. Some went first to the island of Djerba, just off the coast of Libya, and then on to the northern coastal areas of Libya, especially Tripoli, where they lived in a 'Jewish Quarter'. They adopted some of the cultural habits of the local peoples of this area but remained ethnically separate for more than two millennia. In the middle of the nineteenth century the Jewish population of Libya was about 8000, rising dramatically to 34 000 over the next century, mainly as a result of improved health. Following the disruption of North Africa during the Second World War and the establishment of the Jewish State of Israel in 1948, close to 90 per cent of the Libyan Jews took advantage of the 'Law of Return' and emigrated to Israel.

In the early 1970s, Esther Kahana and Harvey Goldberg of the Hebrew University and Hospital in Jerusalem described all the cases of CJD that they could find in Israel (Goldberg *et al.* 1979). There were about two dozen for whom a reasonable amount of data was available. After the Second World War hundreds of thousands of Jews from all over Europe and America had emigrated to Israel, so these scientists were surprised to find that about half of the cases of CJD came from within the group of immigrant *Libyan* Jews. In fact there were more than 30 times as many cases of CJD in this group as would have been expected by chance. Kahana and Goldberg undertook an extensive sociological survey of diet, occupation, kinship, and so on. There seemed to be little difference in cultural habits between the Libyan Jews and those amongst whom they had settled, who were for the most part Jewish immigrants from other parts North Africa, for example Tunisia. For both Libyan Jews and Jews from other parts of North Africa the main source of animal protein was fish, but they also ate lamb and chicken, and both groups ate sheep's heads, including eyeballs and brains. Rabbinical law required that the brain of any animal which was '*mizuna*' (behaving oddly) had to be inspected before it could be eaten. This prevented the brains of sheep with worms or other gross pathology from being eaten. We cannot know whether any of the sheep had scrapie. Scrapie has not been reported in Israel, and there are no data available for Libya. Thus, despite a widespread belief that the Libyan Jews developed CJD from eating the brains and eyeballs of scrapie-affected sheep (Herzberg *et al.* 1974), there was little evidence to support this.

Two of the original 14 Libyan Jews with CJD were related to each other. Three more had parents who were first cousins. This level of consanguinity was common amongst people from North Africa, irrespective of religion. Later, six more cases were found, of which four were familial pairs. There were no familial cases amongst the non-Libyan Jews with CJD, but many of these had limited knowledge of their parents, who had died in Europe during the war. Thus, the impression was gained that the cause of the high incidence of CJD in the Libyan Jews was more likely to be genetic than dietary, but this could not be proved with the limited data available. Molecular genetics was eventually able to establish that the reason for their illness was entirely genetic, and that these patients all belonged to one large, but fragmented, extended family.

One person in Britain

P.S., a 57-year-old married woman, was on holiday at the seaside in August 1954 when she noticed that she was having difficulty controlling her left hand. She had had no previous neurological problems. On her return, P.S. consulted her family doctor about her weak arm and he commented that she also seemed unusually irritable. Within 10 days this irritability had developed into unaccountable 'tantrums'. Her left arm was by now useless and her left leg was beginning to become weak. She was not carrying out her usual household duties and complained of 'muzziness behind the eyes'. Although she denied any specific difficulty with her sight, the doctors noticed that she tended to grope around to find a door handle or to pick up food.

When people lose a perceptual ability because they have damage to a sense organ they are well aware of their disability. For example, people with cataracts are well aware that they cannot see. But when they lose the part of the brain that deals with perception they seem to lose all concept of that ability. Having sustained damage to the visual perceptual parts of the brain, an individual may not only be unable to see, but may be confused about this, and have difficulty explaining what the problem is. When asked why they appear to be having difficulty seeing, such people may make up excuses (for example, that they have lost their glasses, or the lights are dim), or they may try to change the subject (for example, by asking for a cup of tea, or to be taken to the toilet). They may avoid the issue by bursting into tears or losing their temper.

By the time another fortnight had passed, P.S. could not to be left unattended, could not feed or dress herself, and was moderately forgetful of recent events. She was admitted to a general hospital and then rapidly transferred to a neurological hospital in south London. In her early days in hospital, P.S. was to be found lying on her back with her legs extended and her arms pulled up tightly across her chest. This posture is common in people with substantial brain damage. There were occasional rapid jerky movements of the right arm and shoulder, known as myoclonic jerks, which are typical of CJD and arise because the neural balance, which normally keeps muscle tone at an appropriate level is disturbed. P.S. made no response to any visual stimuli, and was judged to be blind, although she denied that this was the case. Her ability to speak and to understand language was well preserved, but simple questions could only be answered after a long pause. She had little to say of her own volition. She could be fed, but only very slowly, and she was not incontinent. Routine hospital investigations failed to reveal any infection or metabolic disorder. A radiograph of the skull was normal. Brain imaging techniques (scans) were not available at that time, but an EEG (electroencephalogram), which measures electrical activity in the brain, showed that brain function was profoundly disturbed. There was a particular rhythmic pattern of slow waves and sharp spikes, which has since come to be regarded as highly characteristic of CJD. Her posture then become progressively more rigid, her head being flexed backward, her arms pulled up with her hands clenched, and her legs beginning to be pulled up towards her body. There were periods when her body went into involuntary rhythmic movements, jerking, or twitching. These symptoms were worse if she was disturbed or handled. After a short period of delirium, in which she appeared to experience frightening hallucinations, P.S. passed into a state of stupor followed by coma. She died 12 weeks after the onset of symptoms.

The post-mortem examination was carried out on the same day. The brain was markedly shrunken, especially the back (occipital cortex), which is involved in visual processing. Microscopical examination revealed severe spongiform change throughout the cortex, together with a loss of neurones, and the proliferation of astrocytes that usually accompanies the loss of neurones. The diagnosis was subacute spongiform encephalopathy. (The patient described in this section is case 4 NSU/Brook Hospital/4709 and is one of a number of cases described in Nevin *et al.* 1960. Her initials are fictitious.)

One family

We were introduced to the world of the transmissible spongiform encephalopathies in 1979 when we drove to Cambridge to have dinner with an old friend who was studying neurology at Addenbrooke's Hospital. Dinner was running a little late because our friend, Jane Adam, had been to see a patient. While the food was being prepared, Jane allowed us to read a preview of her thesis, entitled 'The curse of the W family', submitted as part of the requirement for her Bachelor of Medicine degree and subsequently published in revised form (Adam *et al.* 1982). Not really dinner-party stuff, it catalogued a quiet tale of disease and early death, which had stalked one family in rural Bedfordshire from the end of the nineteenth century. The disease was now claiming the life of another young mother.

When J.C. went for her first appointment at Addenbrooke's Hospital, to see a neurologist about the cramps and 'pins and needles' in her legs and her tendency to stumble when playing tennis, she took her family tree with her. Although her symptoms were very slight and could have been due to any number of causes, she knew that it was likely that she was joining her many relatives in developing a serious and ultimately fatal neurological disease. The family 'curse' had started for sure with great grandma W., who had died of an unspecified neurological disease at the age of 55 years. Sixteen of her 33 direct descendants had subsequently died prematurely of a neurological illness. The most common diagnoses had been multiple sclerosis or spinocerebellar degeneration (a rare, usually hereditary, disease of the spinal cord and cerebellum), but diagnoses of presenile dementia, Parkinson's disease, and brain tumour also appeared on the death certificates.

Some of J.C.'s relatives had been cared for by a general practice in Ampthill in Bedfordshire, and, in 1974, two general practitioners had published a paper describing neurological disease in five other cases in the three generations preceding that of great grandma W., taking the history of the disease back to 1791 (Cameron and Crawford 1974). The tendency to develop disease appeared to run as a dominant trait. (This means that if one person had the disease, half of their children, on average, would eventually become ill, but if a member of the family lived to old age without developing the disease, none of their children would become sick.) If this was true, 58 members of the family, many of whom were still young children, had to be considered to be at some risk. This pattern of disease is seen in Huntington's disease and a few other neurological diseases, but the symptoms in this family did not seem right for any of these other, better known, diseases. The family had only recently begun to appreciate the enormity of the problem, and there was a great deal of anxiety. J.C. was keen to encourage scientific research into the family disease, which is why she had gone to some trouble to prepare the tree, and her efforts proved extremely valuable later on.

Although largely unknown to the general public, inherited neurological diseases are well-known to neurologists and neuropathologists. In the Victorian era, many patients with such diseases were cared for in large institutions, and their familial pattern of disease contributed to the much

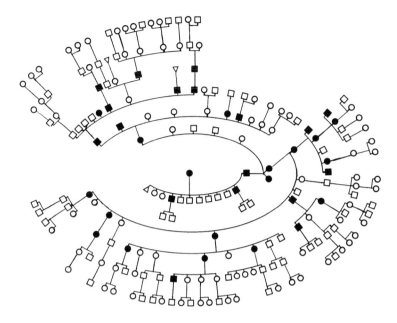

Fig. 4.2 Autosomal dominant inheritance of disease is clearly seen in this large pedigree, in which prion disease is linked to the codon 102 mutation (proline to leucine). The pedigree spans three continents with members in England, North America, and Australia. The filled symbols indicate affected members; circles are females; squares are males; triangles indicate gender unknown.

feared concept of 'hereditary insanity'. However, something singled this family out as being different from other families with inherited neurological diseases. One of great grandma W.'s children had emigrated to the United States, establishing a branch of the family there, and, in 1973, a member of that branch, J.W., had died of a neurodegenerative disease that looked like CJD. Although he had died in Los Angeles on the west coast, brain tissue was sent to Carleton Gajdusek's laboratory near Washington on the east coast. This brain tissue was injected intracerebrally into spider monkeys and squirrel monkeys (both New World species), and into chimpanzees. Within 2 years the monkeys had died of spongiform encephalopathy (Rosenthal *et al.* 1976), although the chimpanzees were reported to be well 7 years later. Transmission to a spider monkey, a chimpanzee, and several guinea-pigs had also been attempted, without success, using the brain of another member of the family, who had died of a similar disease. So J.W. had belonged to a family with an inherited neurological disease, but had died of what was, in the mid-1970s, a 'slow viral' infection. A whole series of questions was raised. Was this family 'inheriting a viral infection'? Or was it inheriting a 'neurological weakness' which rendered members vulnerable to many different types of neurological disease, one case of which was CJD? Was the apparent dominant pattern of inheritance no more than an infection that had a 'hit rate' of about half of the offspring in each family? If so, what were these people doing to pass on an infection, the only known human equivalent of which, kuru, was caused by cannibalism? In Bedfordshire? What kind of a virus was it that could be carried half way round the world to infect someone's offspring 40 years later and yet was not passed to their spouse? Was the virus being passed on to children via the placenta or the mother's milk? This, at least, seemed unlikely, since the disease could appear in a father and some of his offspring without his wife becoming affected. None of the other family members had a diagnosis of CJD, which was defined at that time as a fatal neurological disease with a duration of less than 12 months, with symptoms of dementia and ataxia and a neuropathological picture that included marked spongiform encephalopathy. All the other patients in the family had an illness that lasted for 3 or more years and, in one case, for as long as 10 years. Some of the patients had become demented very early in the course of their illness, so that they had scarcely understood how ill they were, while others had developed only motor symptoms, and had remained lucid and oriented in time and space until the bitter end.

Perhaps the affected members of this family were inheriting an immunological defect that rendered them susceptible to a 'slow virus' which was harmless to most people. For so many of the family members to become ill, this normally harmless virus would have had to be distributed widely throughout the environment. Nevertheless, the hypothesis that the infectious agent was spread as a 'thin veneer' across the whole world was not easily reconciled with the epidemic of kuru, which had had a definite beginning and end. This hypothesis was much favoured by veterinarians interested in scrapie, who had to explain why some sheep got scrapie however hard one tried to separate them from other scrapie-affected sheep. A more elaborate version of the 'thin veneer hypothesis' held that the world was covered in a harmless form of the virus which, when it gained access to the brain, became irreversibly pathogenic (disease-producing). This was supposed to explain why certain people (and sheep) seemed to acquire the disease from nowhere but why, when they had done so, their brains contained large amounts of infectious agent which could easily be used to induce disease experimentally in another animal, or accidentally, as in the case of kuru.

It is difficult to imagine what it is like to be part of the 'W' family. There were times when everything would seem normal for more than a decade, but there were other times when several members of the family were ill at the same time. Because of the illness, family members became more aware of some of their distant relatives than might normally be the case. Everybody grows up knowing more about those of their relatives who are alive than those who have died. So it took quite a lot of effort for J.C. to piece together so much of her family tree. As we have come to know this family over the years, it has become obvious to us that the shared burden of the family illness has brought about a bond of closeness and mutual support that extends to those in the United States as well as in the United Kingdom.

Great grandma W. died sometime near the beginning of the twentieth century at the age of 55 years. Her twin sister died of a similar illness at the same age. The twin's death certificate is issued in her maiden name, suggesting that she had never married and, therefore, had probably not had children. But the twins had other brothers and sisters, some of whom had died in middle age, so it was likely that there were other, as yet untraced, branches of the family. Great grandma W. had eight children and all went well for at least 30 years. But in the 1940s, three of her daughters died, and a son and another daughter died at the end of the 1950s. In the next generation there were nine deaths among 22 cousins between 1968 and 1976. Clearly something was very wrong. An older member of the family told us of his difficulty in deciding what to say to the youngsters in his family. At that time there was nothing that could be done, and no way of predicting who would become ill. (Many families may carry dominant genes which determine early onset cancer, heart disease, and so on, but, unless such a family is both large and close-knit, the pattern may never be discerned. People who carry such genes are not protected from other diseases or accidents, so they may die never knowing of the risk they had been under and that they may have passed to some of their children.) This family member told us of his decision not go to great lengths to explain his concerns about the family illness until his relatives had 'done the young things of life', including marriage and childbearing. There was, he said, time later to start thinking about death and disease. He argued that since each of the young children of his affected relatives had only a 50 per cent chance of themselves becoming ill, many of them would have been worrying unnecessarily. In any case, the value of a life is not determined by its length.

What could be done scientifically to understand the nature of the family disease? The first problem was to decide whether the members of this family all suffered from essentially the same disease. Spongiform encephalopathy had been transmitted from one case (J.W.), although transmission from another case had failed. By this time J.C. was severely ill and she was admitted to Northwick Park Hospital in Harrow, London, for her terminal care. With the family's consent, the post-mortem was carried out by Professor Leo Duchen at the National Hospital for Neurology and Neurosurgery in central London, and we injected brain tissue from J.C. into marmosets (small, captive-bred, New World monkeys) at the Medical Research Council's Clinical Research Centre in Harrow. Nearly 3 years later the marmosets began to show the subtle but characteristic loss of balance and co-ordination that was by now a well-established symptom of transmissible spongiform encephalopathy in monkeys. By coincidence, the first marmoset to show signs of illness was called Daisy, like the first chimpanzee to which kuru was transmitted. The animals were put down before the disease had progressed very far and examination of their brains, again by Leo Duchen at the National Hospital, confirmed the diagnosis (Baker *et al.* 1985). It was our view that the second transmission from affected members of this family made it likely that they had a genetically determined neurodegenerative disease in which an infectious agent was generated *de novo*. In other words it seemed that affected members of the family were *genetically programmed to produce an infectious agent* spontaneously, which could transmit disease experimentally to animals. Indeed, we entitled our report of this work in the *British Medical Journal* 'Experimental transmission of an autosomal dominant spongiform encephalopathy: does the infectious agent originate in the human genome?' A number of British neurologists and veterinarians greeted what they regarded as a somewhat eccentric view with a degree of consternation, and there are still some workers in this field who regard it as ridiculous. However, it was by no means a new concept. James Parry had always maintained that scrapie was a genetically *generated* disease, despite being well aware that the disease could be transmitted by injecting brain tissue from affected sheep into other sheep. And as we described in an earlier chapter, Stan Prusiner, who had been working in San Francisco on scrapie and CJD for several years, had put forward the wholly revolutionary idea that the scrapie agent was associated with and, possibly, comprised solely a novel proteinaceous (protein-containing) infectious particle, which he termed a 'prion' (Prusiner 1982). A little while afterwards, Prusiner and his colleagues were able to demonstrate that this protein was made by the animal or person who was affected, rather than by a virus or other infectious agent, with genes of its own (Oesch *et al.* 1985). This provided a breakthrough in understanding the mechanism by which an inherited gene might lead to a disease that was transmissible. We will discuss this in more detail in Chapter 7.

Gerstmann–Sträussler–Scheinker syndrome (GSS)

In 1981, Colin Masters published a paper in which he pointed out that three suspected CJD patients, whose brains had been used in successful disease transmissions to primates in Gajdusek's laboratory, came from families in which other members had also had neurological disease. In each case the description of the whole family's disease was close to another exceedingly obscure condition known as Gerstmann–Sträussler–Scheinker syndrome or GSS (Masters *et al.* 1981*b*).

In 1936, the three German doctors (two neurologists and a neuropathologist), after whom the disease was named, described a family in which eight young or middle-aged patients had died of a cerebellar ataxia and progressive dementia, lasting several years in each case (Gerstmann *et al.* 1936). The brain of an affected member of this family exhibited some of the hallmarks of CJD, including mild spongiform change and loss of nerve cells, together with the occurrence of a large number of strange, amorphous clumps of an unknown material in the cerebellum, cortex, and brainstem. Colin Masters could find less than two dozen families in the whole world which he thought might have suffered from this exceedingly rare disorder. Three cases came from Japan, one large family came from Germany (in addition to Gerstmann's original family), and one each came from France, Holland, and Scotland. One very large family in the UK, described by Worster-Drought and colleagues (Worster-Drought *et al.*, 1944), had cases in which the brains showed large numbers of strange deposits in the brain, similar to those seen in GSS, but did not show spongiform change. Fifty years after the Worster-Drought family was first described, investigation indicates that they do not suffer from an inherited form of prion disease. They have an illness which is still unique to their family and its cause remains unknown. To the GSS cases published in the literature, Colin Masters was able to add a further seven that had been referred to Gajdusek's laboratory. Transmission had been achieved from three of these cases. Two of the transmitted cases were Japanese. They showed marked spongiform encephalopathy and neuronal degeneration (consistent with CJD), degeneration of the 'white matter' (the fibre tracts within the brain which, because they contain a lot of fat, are white and shiny), which seems to occur mainly in Japanese patients with CJD, and the deposition of plaques (microscopic lumps) of an unknown substance throughout the brain. These two patients had a duration of illness of more than 3 years, which meant that they could not be said to have had 'typical CJD'. The third transmitted case could be said to have had 'typical CJD', except for the appearance of some plaque material in his brain, which was unusual. However, he came from a family in which the average duration of symptoms was too long for CJD, and the spongiform change was frequently not very severe. Where they had been looked for in the brains of his relatives, plaque-like deposits had also been found. This patient was none other than J.W., the grandson of great grandma W. and the cousin of J.C.

J.C.'s brain showed all the hallmarks of this new form of prion disease, the Gerstmann– Sträussler–Scheinker syndrome, or GSS. The spongiform change was marked, and the plaques showed the 'multicentric' shape and distribution within the forebrain and cerebellum, which came to be regarded as definitive of GSS. Samples of her brain were sent for research purposes to laboratories all over the world. Two further members of J.C.'s family have died of the same disease. One showed an atypical and rather limited neuropathological picture, and attempts to prove the diagnosis by transmission to primates were unsuccessful. The second patient, N.D., had all the hallmarks of GSS. He died just a few weeks after his thirty-ninth birthday, having been ill for 2–3 years. After the death of J.C., some 15 years previously, N.D. had assumed a liaising role between members of the W. family and ourselves, and we were much saddened by his death.

Plaques and tangles

In addition to the vacuolated neurones and neurodegeneration, another pathological feature seen in sheep with scrapie were plaques—deposits of an unidentified substance in the brain (Beck *et al.* 1964). This substance was called amyloid. The word amyloid refers to a particular state of a substance, rather than to a particular protein or other chemical substance of which these plaques are made. Originally the term meant 'waxy', but the substance is not a wax. Biochemical analysis suggests that a more appropriate word to describe the constituents of these deposits is 'polymer'. With the use of immunohistochemical techniques, in which tissue is treated with antibodies to different proteins, and then visualized using specific stains attached to the antibodies, it is now possible to show that amyloid can consist of one of several different proteins. Thus the amyloid deposits (plaques) seen in the brains of those who have died from Alzheimer's disease is made of a substance called β-protein, but the amyloid of prion diseases is made of prion protein. This is one of the reasons why CJD, GSS, and some other variants of the disease, which are neither transmissible nor spongiform, are now grouped together as prion diseases. Not all cases of prion disease have amyloid deposits in the brain, so this staining method cannot be used as a simple diagnostic tool for all forms of prion disease. The precise shape of the plaques and the circumstances under which they do, and do not, occur turn out to be very important in understanding the difference between different types of prion disease. These were also crucial pieces of evidence in suggesting that a 'new variant' of CJD (nvCJD) had been seen for the first time in 1994 in Britain, and that cases of nvCJD might be related to the BSE epidemic occurring in Britain.

Immunohistochemical staining for prion protein was only developed in the mid-1980s, so up until that time the identification of amyloid in the brain rested on observing the structure rather than the chemical composition of these deposits. According to Masters *et al.* (1981*b*), about 75 per cent of the brains of kuru victims contained numerous small, star-shaped plaques, which were called kuru plaques, whereas only about 25 per cent of cases of sporadic CJD had kuru plaques. Although the genetic basis that determines whether CJD patients have kuru plaques became clear at a later stage, it is no longer possible to assess what was happening in kuru because there is virtually no tissue left from the original patients, and only a few patients a year are now seen with kuru. It is not even possible to learn much from the genetic make-up of the present-day population of the Foré people of Papua New Guinea. Since so many Foré people died from kuru, it is not clear that the population genetics in the survivors would be the same as it was in the general population at the height of the epidemic. Patients with GSS were defined as those showing a particular type of 'multi-centric' plaque. All patients who have acquired CJD from growth hormone injections have plaques (Ironside 1996*b*).

Elderly patients with CJD or GSS may also have amyloid plaques which stain with antibodies to the β-protein, in addition to prion protein plaques. β-Protein plaques are seen in the brains of patients with Alzheimer's disease, and, to a lesser extent, in the brains of all elderly people. They may be accompanied by other deposits called 'tangles' within the neurones. Tangles are composed of a number of proteins and they indicate that the neurones are no longer functioning properly. Although β-protein amyloid plaques are seen in normal elderly people, they occur in much higher numbers in patients with Alzheimer's disease. Tangles are not seen in normal individuals and are considered indicative of Alzheimer's disease. The β-protein plaques found in some elderly patients with CJD may reflect nothing more than the overlap of the neurodegenerative changes seen in CJD and those seen in normal ageing. In some cases, the plaques are found to contain a mixture of both prion protein and β-protein, suggesting that there may be an interaction between the processes leading to the deposition of the two forms of amyloid. This is important because an understanding of the processes leading to the deposition of one of these forms of amyloid might illuminate the processes leading to the deposition of the other. While CJD is a very rare disease, Alzheimer's disease occurs in a substantial proportion of the elderly population, and, as people live longer (because of the reduction of other diseases), the number of people dying of Alzheimer's disease can be expected to increase substantially. However, while we might learn something about Alzheimer's disease from our studies of the prion diseases, it is not a prion disease, and there is no evidence to suggest that it can be acquired by infection. There is, however, some evidence in animal studies that the process of β-protein amyloid production may be artificially transmissible from one brain to another (Baker *et al.* 1994).

The Indiana pedigree

In the American state of Indiana a number of people were identified in the 1980s who had a disease very similar to GSS (Ghetti *et al.* 1992). Some of these people were closely related to each other while others were not immediately known as relatives. However, investigation of their origins soon showed that they were all members of an extensive, and extensively affected, family or pedigree. By the early 1990s, 10 affected people were being cared for and a further 164 people, mainly children, who carried a 50 per cent risk of developing the illness later in life, had been identified. The pedigree spanned eight generations and there had been a total of 73 affected people. In order to build up this large picture, data on 2226 individuals had to be collected and sifted through. The people in this pedigree clearly suffered from an inherited form of prion disease because their brains were found to contain large numbers of prion protein plaques. But the plaques were also surrounded by deposits of β-protein amyloid, and many of the neurones still remaining contained tangles. There was little spongiform change. Examination of the brains from these patients using only conventional histological stains, which are unable to differentiate between different types of amyloid protein, would have led to a diagnosis of Alzheimer's disease. Attempts to transmit a spongiform encephalopathy to primates, by intracerebral injection of brain tissue from affected members of this pedigree, have been unsuccessful so far. This family appears to be unique in the world, in that no other family has been found that has precisely this pattern of symptoms. However, many other families have similar sorts of symptoms, and these may all be referred to as having variants of GSS, or to be suffering from 'atypical prion disease', a term used to describe new forms of prion disease which do not conform to the precise definition of CJD or GSS. Experimental transmission to animals from cases of atypical prion disease have generally been unsuccessful.

Fatal familial insomnia

In 1992, a new disease, described rather strikingly as 'fatal familial insomnia', appeared on the scene. This was clearly a form of prion disease because PrP^{sc} (the abnormal form of prion protein) could be isolated from brain tissue, but the brain pathology was unusual. The thalamus, a large nucleus (discrete structure) in the centre of the brain, was so markedly affected that it had collapsed and almost disappeared, leaving a large fluid-filled cavity in the middle of the brain. There was some spongiform change, but this was not very severe. The patients' problems consisted of a sleep disturbance which rapidly progressed to a complete inability to sleep or to respond to most sleeping pills. This level of sleep deprivation had profound effects on the patients' mental abilities, and they became confused, disorientated, and showed dream-like, hallucinatory states. In addition, they had profound hormonal disturbances and a breakdown of the neural control of bodily and metabolic functions. In other words, there was a major disturbance of the control of heart rate, blood pressure, temperature, and so on. Eventually they developed motor impairment and memory loss, and lapsed into a stuporous or comatose state before they eventually died.

Amyotrophic CJD

As the new forms of disease described above were shown to be linked to each other, either by successful transmission experiments or, later, by the demonstration of the involvement of prion protein, some diseases previously thought to belong to the group of spongiform encephalopathies were distanced from the group. One such disease was 'amyotrophic CJD'. Amyotrophic means change leading to muscle loss, so this was a disease which comprised the features of degeneration of the motor neurones (the nerve cells which control muscle action), resulting in muscle wasting and paralysis, together with a degenerative process in the brain which was

Table 4.1 Different forms of human prion disease

Creutzfeld–Jakob disease
Symptoms	Dementia, ataxia, myoclonus
Duration	3–12 months
Neuropathology	Spongiform encephalopathy, sometimes PrP plaques
Cause	Usually sporadic, sometimes familial

Kuru, iatrogenic CJD, new variant CJD
Symptoms	Ataxia followed by dementia
Duration	2–24 months
Neuropathology	Spongiform encephalopathy, usually with PrP plaques
Cause	Acquired by contamination

Gerstmann–Sträussler–Scheinker disease
Symptoms	Dementia, ataxia, myoclonus
Duration	1–15 years
Neuropathology	PrP plaques, usually spongiform encephalopathy
Cause	Familial

Fatal familial insomnia
Symptoms	Dementia, failure of autonomic functions, insomnia
Duration	1–15 years
Neuropathology	Spongiform encephalopathy, mainly in the thalamus
Cause	Familial

Atypical prion disease
Symptoms	Dementia, ataxia
Duration	1–15 years
Neuropathology	Usually some PrP plaques, very little spongiform encephalopathy
Cause	Usually familial

associated with dementia. The motor neurones sit within the spinal cord and control muscle groups in the arms, legs, and elsewhere, having received instructions from the motor areas of the brain. Since the brain degeneration frequently resulted in some sponginess in the brain, it was thought that this was a form of CJD. The course of the illness was of rather long duration for CJD but was rapid relative to other forms of neurodegenerative disease. However, since this disease was first described, it has become clear that small areas of sponginess in the cortex may be seen in cases of almost any brain disease that is particularly rapid in its course. The appearance of some sponginess did not in itself imply that these patients must have had CJD, and the failure of transmission studies suggested that they could be safely distanced from CJD, and grouped with other degenerative diseases of the motor neurones. Then a short letter appeared in the medical journal, *Lancet,* announcing that a rhesus monkey which had been injected with brain tissue from a patient with a diagnosis of amyotrophic CJD 9 years earlier had died, and that the monkey's brain had shown the characteristic features of spongiform encephalopathy (Connolly *et al.* 1988). So the possibility of motor neurone pathology in CJD was raised again, although it remains a very rare symptom. Working with this group of diseases is always fascinating because very small pieces of data can have important effects on the way one views a disease, and the perception of what does, and does not, belong in any disease grouping is constantly changing. The most reasonable reconciliation of these disparate pieces of information is that there is a form of motor neurone disease with involvement of the brain's cortex (resulting in dementia), which is unrelated to CJD, but that pathology in CJD occasionally extends to the motor neurones, producing a syndrome which may be difficult to distinguish from other forms of motor neurone disease without exhaustive laboratory tests.

CJD in Great Britain

At the beginning of the 1980s, Professor Brian Matthews, Dr Bob Will, and a small group of investigators in Oxford set out to review the data on as many cases of CJD occurring in the UK during the previous decade as they could find (Will and Matthews 1984; Will *et al.* 1986). They identified 121 neuropathologically confirmed cases and, by examining death certificates and by consulting a large number of neurologists and neuropathologists, found a further 31 probable cases. Wherever possible they obtained hospital notes and examined them in detail. Forty-two cases were rejected as having suffered from some other disease, usually rapidly progressive Alzheimer's disease. Whereas CJD was once frequently missed, it was now sometimes seen when it wasn't there. Cases were found all over England and Wales (the total area surveyed). The majority of patients were between 50 and 75 years old when disease struck and, even when the population was fully corrected for death from other causes, there appeared to be an absence of cases amongst the very elderly. This restricted age range could suggest that CJD really does not occur in the elderly, but it could also suggest that even a disease as rapid and dramatic as CJD could be misdiagnosed when it occurs in the very elderly, perhaps being confused with senile dementia, stroke, or the onset of some other neurological condition followed rapidly by death from pneumonia. In this early survey the overall incidence was found to be about 1 case per year per 3 million of the population. An excess of females was found, but this was not reported in other large surveys. Some geographical clustering was seen, but again this was not confirmed on further investigation. About 6 per cent of cases were found to be familial.

In a 'case-control' survey, which was carried out shortly after the initial surveys were completed (Harries-Jones *et al.* 1988), the past medical and surgical history, diet, occupation, pet ownership, and so on, were compared between cases of CJD and 'controls', patients with a different diagnosis in the same hospital. Since the CJD patients could not answer questions themselves, details had to be obtained from their spouses, partners, or other close relatives. In order to treat each group in the same way, relatives of the 'controls' were also asked the same questions. Apart from a larger number of relatives with some form of dementia amongst the cases (reflecting the familial nature of CJD in a proportion of cases), there were no clear associations between CJD and life events, diet, occupation, or habits, which have been confirmed in further investigations elsewhere. In any case-control study it is more common for 'cases' than 'controls' to report events or factors that they think are relevant to their illness. This is because of a particular psychological stance on the part of the relative or patient making these reports. When trying to come to terms with a serious disease of unknown origin in a relative, someone who is asked about the relative's previous surgery or illnesses is likely to remember every small instance as they 'grasp at straws' to find a reason for the illness. On the other hand, the relative of a person who is well or who has a disease which is common and well understood, is likely either not to think too hard about the minute details of previous events, or to adopt a dismissive 'never done anything odd in his life' attitude. In addition, when a very great many questions are asked in a large survey it is inevitable that some differences will emerge between the 'cases' and the 'controls' which are merely due to chance variation. Thus, only those effects that are large, or that can be confirmed in further analyses, are accepted as being important. When all this was taken into account, there was very little in the lifestyle of the CJD 'cases' to indicate how they came to be ill.

In the course of their investigations, Will and Matthews came across some very curious occurrences. In 1980, a dentist died of CJD in a village in Britain. Looking back through records it was discovered that in the 1960s two people who lived within 250 m of each other, and of the dentist, had also died of CJD. These two people both went to the same general practitioner, but records failed to establish whether they also attended the local dentist, who had used his house as the surgery. The dentist's widow used to have her hair done by the local hairdresser, whose husband had died of CJD. The dentist had a friend who was also a dentist and who worked in a nearby village. Two of *his* patients had also died of CJD. Bob Will remarks that, at this point, he was reluctant to carry out yet further investigations for fear of causing undue alarm (Will 1987). We suspect that geographical clusters such as this usually represent the close genetic relatedness of people who live in stable, rural communities, but we are just as unable to prove this as anyone else is able to demonstrate how these people could have transmitted CJD to each other, having had only limited social contact.

In view of the suspicion that CJD may be acquired by eating meat from an animal with prion disease (either sheep with scrapie or cattle with BSE), or from other exogenous causes, it is important to note that CJD has been found in a lifelong vegetarian who had never had surgery, had never worked on a farm, or in a butcher's shop, and who had never left Britain (Will and Matthews 1981). The CJD literature abounds with stories of this type. They show that when you start to look at the lives of millions of people, you find the most extraordinary coincidences and curious stories. This applies whatever disease is being investigated. They tell us little about the nature of the illness, but they do illustrate the diversity of human experience.

The National CJD Surveillance Unit, Edinburgh

When it became clear that the BSE epidemic in cattle was large, and the possibility that BSE would cause disease in humans could not be ignored, the decision was taken by the UK Department of Health to set up a long-term research project to monitor the occurrence of CJD in the British Isles. It was assumed that a BSE-related disease in people would resemble CJD. Bob Will, now a consultant neurologist at the Western General Hospital in Edinburgh, was appointed to direct the National CJD Surveillance Unit, based at the hospital, and to look after the clinical aspects of the project. His colleague, Jeanne Bell, later to be joined by James Ironside, undertook the neuropathological assessment of the brains of the patients. The CJD Surveillance Unit began its work in 1990. The earlier epidemiological surveys had looked at CJD in England and Wales from 1970 to 1984, so the first job was to fill in the years from 1984 to 1990, and to extend the survey to the rest of the British Isles. The next job was to set up case-control studies which would establish whether new cases of CJD could be related to anything specific in the environment. All neurologists, clinical neurophysiologists, and neuropathologists in the country were contacted regularly and asked to notify the Unit of any patients who might have had CJD. Suspected cases of CJD were visited by a member of the CJD Surveillance Team, and detailed answers to many questions were obtained, usually from a close relative. Control patients were also identified for whom the same detailed answers could be obtained from a relative. Patients were classified as 'definite', 'probable', or 'possible' CJD, according to how many features of the disease they exhibited. Definite cases included those who had a neuropathological diagnosis of spongiform encephalopathy together with either an EEG or a movement disorder which was characteristic of CJD. Probable cases were those having all the clinical symptoms but for which no post-mortem examination was obtained. Even for a disease as alarming as CJD, where it might be expected that relatives are anxious for a definitive diagnosis, a post-mortem examination may not always be carried out, either because the relatives withhold permission, or for some technical or administrative reason. Possible CJD was counted when only historical descriptions were highly suggestive of CJD but where there were inadequate medical records or there was no post-mortem examination. At any one time there would always be some patients in each category, and many patients changed category as time went on. For example, they would change from probable to definite when the post-mortem confirmed the diagnosis. For this reason it is always difficult to say exactly what is happening *now*; allowance always has to made for cases 'in the pipeline'.

Although the aims of the CJD Surveillance Unit were straightforward, there were many logical as well as practical difficulties. Since the original surveys were published, it had become clear that the term 'prion disease' covered a much broader spectrum of clinical presentations than the earlier definitions of CJD. If all cases of prion disease were to be counted, the disease incidence could be much higher than had originally been found for CJD. This might lead to the belief that BSE was causing disease in humans when in fact it was not. If only 'typical' CJD were to be counted, it was possible that, if BSE caused cases of prion disease which differed slightly in presentation from that seen in 'typical' CJD, they might be missed. Should the growth hormone CJD cases, whose clinical picture was not typical of CJD, also be included? How much effort should be made to find out if cases of CJD were familial and, therefore, unlikely to be BSE related? Estimating the numbers of familial cases has a bearing on the interpretation of the whole database. It was anticipated that with all the extra effort to identify as many cases of CJD as possible, the incidence of CJD would be higher than that found in the original surveys. The extent to which the number of familial cases rose could, therefore, be used as a measure of the increased efficiency of ascertainment, which could then be used to decide how much of the higher incidence in sporadic cases could also result from increased efficiency.

Since a definitive diagnosis of CJD depends on post-mortem examination of the brain, it was obvious that this major survey would require extensive neuropathological facilities. The bodies of many suspected cases of CJD are transported to the CJD Surveillance Unit for post-mortem examination, although some examinations are carried out in local hospital departments. In either situation careful safety procedures are necessary, and protocols were drawn up by Jeanne Bell and James Ironside (1993). In addition to all this organizational work, the bringing together of material from a substantial number of cases of CJD from throughout Britain enabled Bell and Ironside to develop more specific histological diagnostic criteria for CJD which, in turn, allowed them to draw up descriptions of the range of neuropathology seen in CJD (Bell 1996; Ironside 1996a).

Not surprisingly, the harder the Surveillance Unit searched, the more cases of CJD they found. There was little that could be done to determine whether the number of cases had been underestimated in the past, but one way of assessing the importance of the higher numbers of CJD cases being seen in Britain, since the advent of BSE, was by comparison with the numbers found in the rest of Europe, where the number of cases of BSE was believed to be minimal. This comparison is still in progress and has required major collaboration between the health services of many European countries. However, it was obvious almost immediately that the number of cases of CJD was rising all over Europe. The number of familial cases was also rising proportionately. All this suggested that CJD had been 'underdiagnosed' throughout Europe until at least the 1990s, and that increased surveillance produced a modest but sustained rise in the number of cases detected.

The Surveillance Unit also found that CJD was much more common in the elderly than had previously been appreciated. Neither an 'environmental' nor 'genetic' explanation of CJD had been able to account for the observation that CJD seemed to be very rare in the elderly. The incidence of sporadic CJD is extremely low below the age of 50, rises steadily until the age of 75, and then drops dramatically, even after correcting for the decline in the size of the population at that age. It is possible that in a very old person, death from pneumonia or a fall (resulting in hip fracture) may occur very early in the course of the disease, so that the underlying illness is not diagnosed. It is also possible that a rapid decline in mental ability in an old person is assumed to be due to a stroke, or senile dementia, without a specific diagnosis being thought necessary. The post-mortem rate is also much lower in the elderly than it is in young people who die unexpectedly. However, when doctors were asked to look for cases of CJD without taking age into account, they found more cases amongst the elderly.

The CJD Unit also found that patients with CJD had consumed higher levels of any kind of meat, especially beef and beef products (according to their relatives), than had the 'controls' (according to their relatives). Did this indicate that CJD was caused by eating meat from infected animals? Or did it merely indicate that the relatives were biased in remembering what had happened in the past, and were attributing blame, according to certain preconceptions about this disease? By the beginning of the 1990s, people in Britain were becoming increasingly aware of a possible link between BSE and CJD, and the idea that all cases of CJD were caught in some way, probably from food, was well-rehearsed by the media. An ingenious way was found to distinguish between these two possibilities. A substantial number of people referred to the CJD Surveillance Unit as possible cases of CJD were found, on post-mortem examination, to have suffered from some other disease. The questionnaires about diet, occupation, and so on were given to the relatives early in the course of the disease, at a time at which both the doctors and the relatives believed that the patient might well be suffering from CJD. It turned out that these 'not-CJD' cases had consumed just as high levels of meat and meat products and were just as likely to have carried out meat-related work (according to their relatives) as the confirmed CJD cases. This strongly suggests that the differences between the CJD patients and the controls was due to psychological factors in the relatives rather than to any real difference in exposure to animals, meat, or meat products.

Four farmers and a couple of youngsters

In 1993 two letters appeared in the *Lancet* reporting the occurrence of CJD in two dairy farmers in Britain, both of whom had had BSE in their herds (Davies *et al.* 1993; Sawcer *et al.* 1993). Both men were middle aged, and their clinical disease and neuropathological picture looked characteristic of sporadic CJD. The time between the occurrence of BSE in their herds and the onset of their illness was about 4 years for one farmer, but less than 1 year for the other. In the second case, the time difference was too short for the farmer to have acquired the disease from his affected cows. There are more than 100 000 people in Britain employed in dairy farming so the occurrence of two cases of CJD in that group might not be remarkable. Not much attention was given to these two cases, or, indeed, to a third affected farmer, until 1995, when a fourth farmer was reported to have developed CJD (Smith *et al.* 1995). This person was also middle aged and had 'typical' CJD. Despite attempts to argue that the incidence of CJD in farmers was similar in Europe to that seen in Britain (Delasnerie-Laupretre *et al.* 1995), the media and the general public were by now alarmed. This alarm was heightened by the report of CJD in two British teenagers (Bateman *et al.* 1995; Britton *et al.* 1995). An extensive debate took place in the *British Medical Journal* (vol. 311, pp. 1415–21, 1995) between those who thought that these cases were BSE-related and those who thought either that they were not, or, at least, that there was no possible way of knowing whether they were or were not. Sheila Gore, a statistician working at the Institute of Public Health in Cambridge, provided a mathematical analysis based, in part, on estimates of the numbers of farmers and farming-related workers in Britain, and came to the conclusion that 'Taken together, cases of Creutzfeldt–Jakob disease in farmers and young adults are more than happenstance.' Paul Brown, on the other hand, commented that 'Statistical analysis will not yet be helpful in our evaluation of these cases, even if the observed occurrence can be shown to exceed significantly the expected occurrence in adolescents and farmers, because the power of statistics when dealing with so few cases is not compelling.' Strictly speaking, the power of statistics does take into account the sample size that is being assessed, but when the number of cases is extremely small it is still likely that the numbers observed, even if not random, are not due to the factor that is being assessed. It should be remembered that these cases were being assessed against an estimate of the number of farmers in Britain. If that estimate was inaccurate or misleading, no amount of mathematical manipulation of the data could strengthen the argument.

In 1996, it became clear that the two teenagers with CJD were but the first of several young people in Britain to die of CJD. These new cases showed a clinical and pathological picture which was so unlike sporadic CJD that they were termed new variant CJD, and it was supposed that they had acquired their disease from eating beef products contaminated with BSE (Will *et al.* 1996). Whether or not this is so, and how it might have come about, will be discussed in detail in Chapter 9. At this point it is necessary only to consider that the farmers did not have the clinical presentation or the neuropathological picture of new variant CJD. So, if it is supposed that the teenagers' disease was BSE-related, this makes it unlikely that the farmers' illness was also BSE-related.

Prion disease today

Apart from a few scientists with ideological objections, most people working in this field now regard CJD as one of a group of diseases which collectively can be termed human prion diseases. They are grouped together, and separated from all other diseases, by virtue of the involvement of the abnormal form of prion protein (PrP^{sc}) in pathogenesis (the development of disease). CJD is defined as a dementing illness of less than 12 months' duration with a neuropathological picture that includes spongiform encephalopathy. When it is attempted, these cases are almost always transmissible to primates by intracerebral injection of brain material. CJD and kuru are similar, except that, in kuru, dementia is a late feature in the course of disease development and the neuropathology is more likely to include amyloid plaques containing prion protein. Gerstmann–Sträussler–Scheinker disease (GSS) has a much longer time course and the deposition of prion protein plaques can be severe. Fatal familial insomnia (FFI) is diagnosed where the symptoms are concerned primarily with the control of sleep and other bodily functions, and the pathology is confined largely to the thalamus. Any other neurodegenerative disease in which the accumulation of PrP^{sc} can be demonstrated in brain is a prion disease but, if it lacks the usual hallmarks of spongiform encephalopathy and does not transmit to primates, it is likely to be called 'atypical prion disease' (APD).

It is now generally accepted that there are three separate ways in which human prion disease can occur. Acquired cases are those in which the person has been contaminated with PrP^{sc} from another human being, either by ingestion, as in the case of kuru, or by medical accident, usually following treatment with contaminated human growth hormone or dura mater. Where the contamination is intracerebral, the incubation time can be as short as 18 months. When the contamination is peripheral, the incubation time can be from 4 to 40 years. Whether new variant CJD has been acquired from BSE-related material is not yet proven, but seems likely. Sporadic CJD occurs in later middle age and is not associated with any known antecedent events. Such cases account for about 85 per cent of the total at present and are thought to be wholly idiopathic (internally generated rather than precipitated by any external event). Familial cases also have an onset in middle age and their cause is wholly genetic. Most of these cases of human prion disease which are not CJD are familial. The perceived incidence of human prion disease tends to rise when strenuous efforts are made to find it. Many countries now record an incidence of about 1–2 cases per million of the population per year. Cases of human prion disease are still extremely rare, but they are important because they are invariably fatal and potentially hazardous in a way that cannot easily be rectified. They also involve a unique pathological mechanism which is unlike that seen in any other conventional infectious disease and is, therefore, of great interest to biologists. More papers are published on the subject of prion disease than there are people who suffer from it. Many scientists who work in the field, ourselves included, would admit to being addicted to trying to understand it.

5

In the laboratory

Following the demonstration in 1936 that scrapie was experimentally transmissible, there was little progress in scrapie research for many years. Agricultural research during the 1940s was seriously affected by the Second World War, and science took a long time to recover from the resulting economic and academic disruption. Although some important work was carried out in sheep, there were few advances in understanding the basic science of scrapie in the post-war period.

The revival of interest in scrapie

The 1960s saw the beginning of a new era in scrapie research. Hadlow's letter to the *Lancet* in 1959 had drawn attention to the similarities between scrapie and kuru and opened up scrapie research to encompass human disease (leading to the experimental transmission of kuru and CJD to primates). In 1961, Dick Chandler of the Institute of Animal Health in Compton, Berkshire, succeeded in transmitting scrapie to mice, with a relatively short incubation period (Chandler 1961). This did not just indicate that scrapie could affect other species; it provided the possibility of doing experiments in large numbers of animals in the laboratory rather than in a few sheep at a time. Some time later, mouse-adapted scrapie was transmitted to hamsters, which have somewhat larger brains than mice, allowing the production of larger amounts of infectious tissue. Incubation periods in hamsters are often even shorter than in mice, making transmission experiments much quicker to carry out. These sorts of changes in technique can often have as big an effect on scientific progress as some important scientific insight.

At this time it was assumed that scrapie was caused by some sort of virus, although it was always recognized as being a peculiar kind of virus. This did not matter much because there were other peculiar viruses, including the 'slow viruses', a name first used by an Icelandic scientist, Bjorn Sigurdsson, to describe the infectious agent that caused visna-maedi disease in sheep and which later turned out to be a retrovirus. This group of viruses, which includes the human immunodeficiency virus (HIV), causes diseases that have very long incubation periods from exposure to overt illness. It was also recognized that some viruses could become latent (inactive) within an infected individual and flare up in disease many years later. Thus, shingles is a late manifestation of latent infection with the virus that causes chickenpox in childhood, and subacute sclerosing panencephalitis is a chronic brain disease (occasionally mistaken for long-duration prion disease) which occurs as a late effect of measles infection.

What kind of an infectious agent caused scrapie?

In attempting to identify the agent (infectious particle or virus), scientists carried out many experiments to assess its properties. First, it was very difficult to destroy. For example, it could survive indefinitely in dead tissue preserved in formaldehyde solution, and was not destroyed by boiling, or by some other methods of sterilization, which would inactivate most conventional viruses and bacteria. This resistance to inactivation had clear safety implications and the agent acquired a frightening reputation, especially amongst scientists who were used to viruses and bacteria being fragile and easily destroyed. Viruses, in particular, do not usually survive for long outside living cells. The second problem was to isolate the agent from the infected tissue. The usual repertoire of biochemistry laboratory techniques was used. In brief, the infected tissue (in the case of the agents of spongiform encephalopathy this usually means brain tissue) is homogenized in a blender to produce a mush. Various 'fractions' can be produced from this homogenate by extracting with different chemical solutions, or by spinning the homogenate in a centrifuge and separating the fractions according to the density of the material in those fractions. The intention is to prepare fractions in which the infectious agent is concentrated. Every time an experiment was done to enrich fractions for infectivity (or to try to destroy infectivity), the results of the manipulation had to be tested by injecting the fractions into mice and waiting up to a year to see whether they became sick. Thus, many experiments had to be started before the results of the previous experiments were known. The work was unbelievably tedious, appealing only to a certain type of scientist. The infectious agent turned out to be very 'sticky' and to adhere to bits of cell membrane in the homogenate. It could, however, be partly separated out by filtration. Tissue homogenate could be passed through ever finer filters until the infectivity could no longer be found in the fluid that passed through the filter. The agent was estimated to have a diameter slightly bigger than 30 nanometres (a nanometre is 1 millionth of a millimetre), which was small even for a virus. Viruses range in size from the roughly spherical virus particles causing poliomyelitis (about 30 nanometres in diameter) up to the elongated virus particles causing disease in tobacco plants (about 300 nanometres long by 15 nanometres wide). Viruses can be destroyed by irradiation, which breaks up their genetic material, but irradiation did little to the scrapie agent. Having concentrated the infectious agent by filtration, and other methods of separation, from tissue debris, scientists should have been able to see particles of the agent under the most powerful electron microscopes that were then coming into use. Sometimes particles were seen, and even in the 1990s, new particles apparently only occurring in scrapie-infected tissue were seen and a great deal of excitement was generated. Only after more study, however, did it become clear that either these particles are also seen in uninfected tissue or they could not be found again and the trail went cold once more.

Not only could researchers not find the infectious agent by these measures, the infected animal also did not seem to 'notice' that it was infected. When a foreign protein that is part of an infectious agent (either a virus or a bacterium) enters the body, the body's immune system swings into action, recognizes the protein as 'non-self' and produces antibodies that attack the foreign protein and contribute to the infection being overcome. (The same process is responsible for the 'rejection' of transplanted hearts and kidneys, and is the reason why transplant patients have to take drugs that suppress their immune systems. Sometimes the body produces antibodies that target the body's own proteins, leading to autoimmune diseases such as myasthenia gravis, rheumatoid arthritis, and, possibly, multiple sclerosis.) No scrapie-specific antibodies were found in infected animals. This added to the mysterious character of the scrapie agent; it crept around the body like some ghost, casting no shadow.

By the early 1960s, James Parry, working at the Nuffield Institute of Medical Research in Oxford, had concluded that the pattern of occurrence of natural scrapie was consistent with scrapie being a recessive disease, and that, *despite being experimentally transmissible,* the disease in sheep was wholly genetic (Parry 1962). This was heresy since, by this, he meant that a gene (or genes) was causing disease directly, rather than making the animal susceptible to catching disease from the environment. This view was hotly contested by John Stamp and Alan Dickinson of the Moredun Research Institute in Edinburgh (Dickinson *et al.* 1965). They were well aware that scrapie tended to occur in ewes and their lambs, but attributed this either to genetic susceptibility to the infectious agent in the environment, or to the direct transfer of the infectious agent through the placenta into the offspring. This disagreement went beyond the limits of 'rigorous scientific debate' and became very personal. Twenty years later, and from as far away as Papua New Guinea, Michael Alpers felt drawn to comment on 'the petty squabbles' in his foreword to Parry's book, entitled *Scrapie disease in sheep*, published in 1983. Even today there is still a feeling of opposing 'camps' in scrapie research, which does no credit to either side.

Why the agent is not a virus

There are many different types of viruses but they share common features that distinguish them from other types of organism. A full discussion of virus structure and replication is beyond the remit we have set ourselves, so we will limit our story to some basic facts, enough to set in context the arguments against the scrapie agent being a virus.

Most viruses, those that cause disease in animals and humans, consist of a core of nucleic acid (either DNA or RNA), surrounded by a coat made up of protein. Viruses gain access to the body in different ways. Some, like those that cause colds and influenza, are shed in droplets during coughing and sneezing and are breathed in by an unfortunate bystander, who, after a short incubation period, will develop disease. Many millions of virus particles will enter the respiratory tract of the victim and will attach themselves to the appropriate target cells (the linings of the airways, etc.). The virus will enter the cell, and, using its own nucleic acid core as a template and its own proteins as enzymes, will make use of the cell's mechanisms to make more copies of its own nucleic acid and its coat proteins. In other words, the viral nucleic acid (the viral genome) contains all the information necessary to direct the synthesis of exact copies of the virus. Many millions of virus particles will be produced before the cell splits apart, releasing them and allowing them to go on to infect other cells. The body's immune system will be actively trying to generate antibodies to the viral coat proteins in an attempt to inactivate the virus, and will usually win. Most infections of this sort are of limited duration. Other viruses have evolved different strategies for survival and replication. A good example is the human immunodeficiency virus (HIV) which causes AIDS (acquired immune deficiency syndrome). This is a retrovirus, having a core of RNA. It is transmitted usually by blood (or other bodily fluids) to blood contact, and targets the cells of the immune system. Having entered a cell, the viral nucleic acid codes for a *reverse transcriptase* enzyme which makes a DNA copy of the viral RNA. This DNA is then incorporated into the genomic DNA of the cell, becoming, in effect, part of the cell's genome. Virus particles are generated as part of the cell's normal synthetic mechanisms, and a chronic infection is set up which slowly destroys the body's immune system.

Viruses come in all shapes and sizes. Some, like the plant viroids, have very simple nucleic acid genomes and no coat protein, while others carry enough genetic information to specify a large number of protein products. The important thing to remember is that viruses have an independent nucleic acid genome; independent, that is, of the host genome. Because this genome is used to direct the replication, or copying, of the virus, and because errors sometimes creep into the copying process, virus particles will occasionally be produced with a slightly different genome. These copying errors are the basis of mutations. When the replication process throws up virus particles with slightly different characteristics, these mutant strains may actually better survive the efforts of the immune defences and replicate better than the original strain.

The evidence against the scrapie agent being a virus is essentially of two kinds. The first is the inability to find a virus. Only the very largest of the viruses can be seen by the most powerful of the conventional light microscopes. With the development of the electron microscope (referred to universally as the EM) in the 1950s and 1960s, the world of the small viruses came into view. Using various EM techniques, in combination with those of X-ray diffraction, scientists unravelled the beautiful and complex structure of viruses. Virus particles could be captured on film, bursting forth from infected cells in their millions, or making a furtive exit ('budding off') from the cell's membrane. Yet, despite these major advances in virology, no virus particle unequivocally associated with spongiform encephalopathy has ever been seen. Unequivocally, because there have been reports of 'virus-like' structures from time to time, but these findings are often not replicated. Here, of course, we use the term replicate in the sense of a different scientist being able to repeat the work of another and to confirm the results! Pawel Liberski, a distinguished electron microscopist from Lodz in Poland, has consistently seen what he describes as tubulofilamentous particles in the brains of animals and humans with spongiform encephalopathy (Liberski

1990). While others have seen such particles there is no general consensus on what they are, and not everyone can find them. Similarly, Heino Diringer in Berlin, a fervent believer in a scrapie virus (Diringer *et al.* 1994), has recently seen particles in EM pictures of scrapie-affected hamster brain tissue and in brain tissue from patients with CJD. Although these particles are very small, he thinks they may be virus particles; again this is not generally accepted. In Britain, Harash Narang (1996) has also reported finding tubulofilamentous structures in the brains of BSE-affected cattle, although he would no doubt agree that his findings have been treated with much scepticism.

Another approach in the search for direct evidence for a virus involves extracting all the nucleic acid from a sample of normal brain, purifying it by conventional biochemical means, and separating it into fractions according to size, and then doing the same with the nucleic acid from scrapie-infected brain. If there is a substantial amount of scrapie-specific nucleic acid in the infected cells, there should be a difference in the fractional distribution. There are variations on this methodology, but they all involve looking for a nucleic acid or a nucleoprotein (nucleic acid combined with a protein) which is found only in scrapie-infected brains and not in uninfected brains. Suffice it to say that there is no accepted evidence of such infection-specific nucleic acid.

The second kind of evidence against scrapie agent being a virus is the inability to destroy infectivity. Most of these experiments have focused on the nucleic acid necessary for conventional viral replication. Nucleic acids are easily destroyed by specific enzymes such as ribonucleases and deoxyribonucleases which 'chew' up RNA and DNA, respectively. Yet treatment of infectious fractions from scrapie-infected animal brain with these enzymes does not reduce its infectivity. Similarly, irradiation with ultraviolet light of a specific wavelength, or heating with harsh chemicals which destroy nucleic acids are without effect in reducing infectivity. Some known viruses can survive some of the treatments thrown at them and there are plausible explanations for this. In some cases, for example, the complex coat proteins may prevent the degrading enzymes from gaining access to the core nucleic acid. However, no conventional virus is resistant to all those treatments that the scrapie agent can survive.

Most scientists would agree that there is no good evidence for the spongiform encephalopathies being caused by a conventional virus, and, further, that there is no good evidence for the existence of a scrapie-specific nucleic acid within infectious fractions prepared from brains.

Virinos and other hypotheses

There has rarely been a shortage of ideas about what the scrapie agent might be. At the turn of this century scrapie was thought to be caused by a small parasitic animal in the sheep's brain. Then, as we have seen, it was widely held to be a 'filterable' virus. By the 1960s a number of scientists were beginning to argue that the agent might be a 'replicating protein' (Griffiths 1967; Pattison and Jones 1967). These early suggestions that the agent might be composed of just protein are interesting because they recognize that the agent could not be a virus. They failed insofar as they were not followed up in experimental studies, perhaps because the necessary techniques were not available at the time. The concept of 'replicating protein' was, and remains, heretical within our understanding of the basis of molecular biology, in which proteins are made under the control of nucleic acid. None the less these early hypotheses recognized that scrapie was different from other forms of infection and had the courage to put forward radical suggestions. Various other theories were advanced, suggesting that the agent contained some sort of free-floating host nucleic acid, together with other material from the host. These ideas were precursors of the concept of retroviruses, which, as we have seen, can insert their nucleic acid into the genetic material of the host and behave sometimes like a gene and sometimes like a virus. This idea went some way to explaining the genetics and transmissibility of scrapie, but now specific tests can demonstrate that the scrapie agent is not a retrovirus.

A view held in high regard by some scientists for almost 20 years is that the agent consists of an informational nucleic acid (probably DNA) which, although big enough to act as a template for its own replication, is too small to code for protein synthesis, and which escapes detection in the infected host by using host-made protein as a coat. This hypothetical agent has been christened a 'virino' (Dickinson and Outram 1979), a sort of 'wolf in sheep's clothing'. The suggestion was that the infected host (the sheep) would recognize the protein coat as being made of sheep material and would not mount an immunological attack on the infecting 'wolf' within. The hypothesis was later modernized by supposing that the host protein was prion protein. This meant that much of the data on the involvement of prion protein in the characteristics of disease, for example the effect of the prion protein gene in the host on incubation time, could be accommodated by supposing that the agent had properties which were due partly to the effect of the virino nucleic acid and partly due to effect of the host prion protein. In particular, it was supposed that strain characteristics were determined by information in the virino nucleic acid but that almost everything else was determined by the protein coat. According to Dickinson and Outram, the authors of the early formulation of this hypothesis, the virino belongs to a class of agents 'which (by analogy with neutrinos) are small immunologically neutral particles with high penetration properties but needing special criteria to detect their presence'. The analogy is weak, however. The existence of neutrinos was proved by Frederick Reines and Clyde Cowan in 1956; virinos remain hypothetical.

Scrapie-associated fibrils (SAFs)

Pat Merz, an electron microscopist working at Staten Island, New York, made a discovery at the beginning of the 1980s which was to be of great practical help in the diagnosis of prion disease. She and her colleagues found that if tissue containing infectious agent was subjected to biochemical procedures that included treating the tissue with detergents, a particular protein would precipitate out as fibrils (very small fibres) which could be seen using an electron microscope (Merz *et al.* 1981). These fibrils were initially extracted from rodent-adapted scrapie-infected brain and were called scrapie-associated fibrils, or SAFs. If uninfected tissue was subjected to the same processing, SAFs could not be seen. Was this the infectious agent? Not quite. It was soon to be shown that SAFs were made of prion protein, but it was also clear that these fibrils were actually assembled during the chemical treatment of the tissue and that they did not exist in the original infected brains in a fibrillar form which could be seen in the EM. None the less, there was a close association between SAFs and infectivity since tissue fractions from which large amounts of SAFs could be prepared were also found to contain high levels of infectivity. The demonstration that SAFs could be prepared from a tissue sample became diagnostic of prion disease in the animal, or person, from which the tissue had been taken. Unfortunately, the absence of SAFs was not proof of the absence of prion disease. SAFs may not be detectable in tissue preparations from those human cases described as having atypical prion disease, and cows or sheep who are incubating prion disease will not yield SAFs until near the time of onset of symptoms.

The discovery of PrP27–30

At about the same time as the work on SAFs was being done in New York, scientists in Stan Prusiner's lab in San Francisco were attempting to purify the infectious agent from the brains of hamsters with rodent-adapted scrapie. Using the biochemical fractionation techniques referred to earlier, and by determining infectivity in the various fractions by tedious transmission experiments, they were able to concentrate most of the infectivity in one fraction. This allowed them to determine what was in that fraction but was not in an equivalent fraction prepared from uninfected brain tissue. The answer was a protein. One feature of this protein made it easy to find but difficult to work on. As part of the biochemical processing, the brain homogenate was treated with a particular enzyme, proteinase K, which digests (breaks up) proteins. Extracts from the infected brain contained a protein fragment that was resistant to proteinase K digestion and which was not seen in the normal brain. This very large residue, subsequently called PrP27–30, which was actually the greater part of the infection-associated protein, was left behind after this treatment. PrP27–30 retained some infectivity but the fact that it was so insensitive to further treatments meant that it was difficult to analyse further because it was, by now, an insoluble substance. The detection of PrP27–30 (where 'PrP' can be taken to mean *protease-resistant protein* and '27–30' refers to its molecular weight) did, however, become another important diagnostic tool because its presence was always indicative of infectivity in the original tissue. This was the protein christened prion protein by Prusiner.

Where did PrP27–30 come from?

Many scientists have contributed to the molecular biological analysis of prion protein, and it would be invidious to name only some and the biochemical techniques they used to study prion protein. Prusiner (1992) has provided a good overview of the discovery of prion protein, and the techniques required to study prion protein are described in Baker and Ridley (1996). Very technical aspects of the molecular biology of prion protein are discussed in Prusiner (1996).

Having produced a relatively pure extract of a protein, scientists were able to work out the amino acid sequence of at least part of the protein. Proteins vary enormously in the order of occurrence of amino acids in their primary structure. If the order of amino acids in even a fairly short length of this primary structure is determined, it will be unique for that protein. The reader might need reminding here that in normal protein synthesis, the information 'encoding' the order or sequence of amino acids in the protein is carried within the sequence of DNA bases in the gene for that protein. The gene sequence is transcribed into a complementary RNA (messenger RNA) which acts as the template for the protein synthetic mechanisms of the cell to make the protein. It is possible to trace this route backwards (we will gloss over these techniques). When the scientists had worked out the partial amino acid sequence of PrP27–30, they were able to synthesize a complementary DNA (cDNA) based on that sequence. Using this cDNA, which exactly complements a unique sequence within the DNA of the gene, they were able to identify the gene encoding PrP27–30. This is the PrP gene.

The PrP gene

It soon became clear that the gene encoding prion protein was not a viral gene but a surprisingly ordinary gene in the host. Some genes are made up of bits of DNA spread out across part of a chromosome, and slightly different proteins can be made from one gene by incorporating only parts of the whole sequence in the protein. This was not the case for the PrP gene. The PrP gene was found to be located on chromosome 20 in humans and on chromosome 2 in mice.

The PrP gene has been identified in a wide range of mammals and birds, and genetic sequences similar to those in the PrP gene have been found in fruit flies and yeast, suggesting that there is little variation in the gene across different species. This is referred to by saying that the gene is 'highly conserved'. During the copying process that goes on when genes replicate, there is a low possibility that mistakes will occur and that the gene will then code for a protein with a slightly different amino acid sequence. If these mistakes, or mutations, are not important for the function of the protein, they will be copied across many generations and, as evolution progresses, the gene will become very varied. If the protein has a very precise function, small changes in the gene are likely to mean that the protein will not function and that any animal carrying that mutant gene will die. The fact the PrP gene is highly conserved across species that diverged millions of years ago implies that the function of prion protein is very important. But it is one of the many puzzles of prion disease that the normal function of prion protein is not known and that it is possible to make mice lacking the

PrP gene, which live a fairly healthy life. That the gene should be so highly conserved, but not essential to existence, is paradoxical.

Unless the rate at which a protein is being broken down is known, it is very difficult to work out how much of it is being made. However, the level of protein messenger RNA (mRNA) can be measured and this gives a good estimate of the rate of protein synthesis. By measuring levels of prion protein mRNA it could be shown that prion protein was being synthesized in many tissues throughout the body, but that the greatest amount was made in the brain and spinal cord. This was interesting because in an infected animal the brain and spinal cord contain the greatest amount of infectivity at the end-stage of the disease, but it was somewhat surprising to find that the amount of PrP produced was the same in both infected and uninfected animals. How could this be, since PrP27–30 was found in infected but not in uninfected animals? In other words, both normal and scrapie-infected animal brains are producing similar levels of prion protein mRNA and yet PrP27–30, which was increasing in line with the infectivity in scrapie-infected animals, could not be extracted from normal brains.

PrP27–30 had been found by digesting infected tissue with proteinase K. Without this step in the analytical procedure the PrP was found to be a larger protein called PrP33–35. PrP33–35 was abundant in the brain of infected and uninfected animals. What appeared to be happening was that the normal form of PrP was being modified in some way in infected animals so that, whereas normal PrP was easily broken down, the disease-modified form could only be broken down partially, to leave a residue of indestructible PrP27–30.

What was PrP?

The demonstration that PrP was coded for by a host gene disposed of the heretical idea that a disease-associated protein was capable of replicating itself without recourse to DNA. Some scientists took the view that PrP was just a host protein that was in some way implicated in the disease process in the host, but that it had little to do with the infectious agent; some scientists thought that PrP might be a normal host protein that was hijacked by the infectious agent and incorporated into the infectious particle (perhaps as a coat around the agent-specific nucleic acid); and some thought that the change in the host protein from the normal to the abnormal form was the crux of the disease and that no other infectious elements were involved. The problem for the adherents of this latter view was to explain how, and under

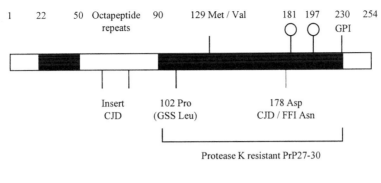

Fig. 5.1 This schematic of the human prion protein molecule illustrates some of the features of the primary structure. The molecule is 250 amino acids long, although the first 22 and the last 24 amino acids are removed from the protein during post-translational processing. A glycosylphosphatidyl inositol (GPI) molecule is attached at position 230 and the prion protein is attached by this to the membrane of the cell. Glycosylated side-chains (oligosaccharides) can attach at either one or both of positions 181 and 197. The protease-resistant core of the molecule lies approximately between positions 90 and 230. Between amino acids 50 and 90 there are five repeats of an octapeptide (eight amino acid) sequence. Position 129 can be filled by either a methionine (Met) or valine (Val) (this is the common polymorphism). Insertions consisting of extra octapeptide repeats are usually associated with CJD or APD. The first mutation to be linked to human prion disease is at position 102, which is normally occupied by the amino acid, proline (Pro). In GSS the proline is replaced by a leucine (Leu). In normal individuals position 178 is occupied by aspartic acid (Asp). If this amino acid is replaced by asparagine (Asn), the resulting prion disease will present as FFI if there is a methionine at position 129, and as CJD if there is a valine at position 129. More than 20 different mutations in the prion gene can lead to prion disease.

what circumstances, the normal form of PrP (now called PrP^c where the ^{c} stands for cellular) was changed into PrP^{sc} (the disease-associated abnormal form, where ^{sc} stands for scrapie) and to explain how this conversion could be transferable from one animal to another.

The deposition of PrP in the brain

Shortly after the discovery of SAFs, scientists in Prusiner's laboratory reported that the PrP, which they had partially purified, formed rod-like structures. These structures were called prion rods, and for a while there was sharp debate as to whether SAFs and prion rods were essentially the same thing. Since antibody studies soon established that SAFs, like prion

rods, were made of PrP, and the structural differences between SAFs and
prion rods were no more than might have been expected from slightly
different methods of preparation, these differences became unimportant. It
has been remarked that 'a scientist would rather use another scientist's
toothbrush than use his terminology' and this seems to have been what
happened in this case. When these rods or fibrils were stained with a dye
called Congo Red and viewed under a low-power microscope, using
polarized light, they glowed either orange or green, depending on the
rotation of the polarized light. This physicochemical property is known as
birefringence and is characteristic of a type of polymer called an 'amyloid'.
This led the scientists back to the brains of patients and animals with prion
disease. As we have already mentioned, the brains of some patients with
prion disease had numerous small plaques of unknown substance deposited
in the tissue. These plaques were similar to (but subtly different from) the
plaques which were an important diagnostic feature of Alzheimer's disease.
Both types of plaque were made of an amyloid substance, as demonstrated
by Congo Red birefringence, but the term amyloid merely implies that the
substance has a certain physical property, rather than that it is composed of
a particular chemical. That PrP^{sc} could form an amyloid substance in a test
tube suggested that the amyloid plaques in the brains of patients with prion
disease might actually be made of PrP. Using immunohistochemical
techniques, in which an antibody specific to PrP and carrying a coloured
marker is used to label thin sections of brain tissue, it was possible to
demonstrate that the amyloid plaques in brain tissue of patients with prion
disease were made of deposits of PrP. This meant that it was also possible to
say that if abnormal structures in a brain section were found to stain with
antibodies to PrP then that person, or animal, had a prion disease.

Separation of infectivity from amyloid

When neuropathologists saw PrP plaques in the brain of a patient who had
died of prion disease, were they looking at the infectious agent which had
killed the patient? Not quite. Only about 15 per cent of cases of CJD had
any PrP plaques in their brain; only aggregations of protein that are large
enough to have some visible structure will be detectable by Congo Red
birefringence and therefore be definable as amyloid. So, the majority of
cases of CJD could not be said to have PrP-amyloid in their brains. There
was also the curious observation, particularly in human prion disease, that
those cases dying within a few weeks of illness onset had the most severe

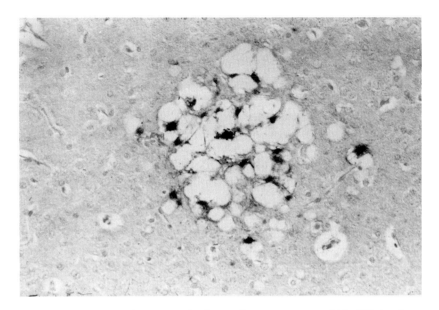

Fig. 5.2 Prion protein deposits in the brain of a marmoset to which BSE has been experimentally transmitted (magnification ∼ 400). The dark patches are aggregations of prion protein around which spongiform change can also be seen. (Photograph by G. A. H. Wells.)

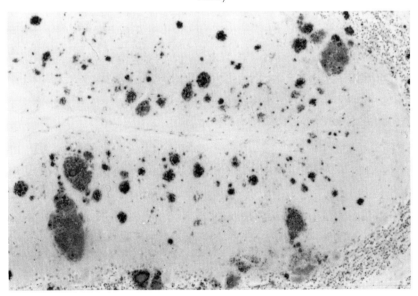

Fig. 5.3 Prion protein deposits in the cerebellum of a patient with prion disease (GSS) (magnification ∼ 150). Even under very low-power magnification, large deposits of prion protein can be seen as dark blobs. (Photograph by J. W. Ironside.)

spongiform encephalopathy and were most likely to be experimentally transmissible to primates; they were also the cases least likely to have PrP-amyloid plaques. Where PrP-amyloid plaques and spongiform encephalopathy did occur in the same brain, it was quite likely that each would occur most extensively in different parts of the brain. One interpretation would be that during the disease process, normal prion protein, PrP^c, is converted into the protease-resistant form, PrP^{sc}, and that, while the body normally destroys PrP^c as part of its 'turnover' of chemicals, it had difficulty in destroying PrP^{sc}. If the body could not break down PrP^{sc} at all then the PrP^{sc} would remain in its most infectious form, and would rapidly kill the host. If PrP^{sc} could be partially broken down into a smaller protein fragment, such as PrP27–30, this chemical could form an amyloid aggregation in the brain tissue. The brain would then gather it up into deposits or 'rubbish dumps' which would eventually become big enough to be seen under a low-power microscope. Being able partially to inactivate PrP^{sc} would allow the patient to live longer; PrP-plaques, although providing evidence of the occurrence of a disease process, might actually reflect the body's ability to cope with the disease to some extent. Analysis of the brains of some patients with familial prion disease of long duration has shown that the PrP-amyloid, which is extensive in their brains, consists of even shorter lengths of prion protein (for example, PrP11, which has a molecular weight of 11 kilodaltons). These familial cases have mutations in the PrP gene suggesting that the unusual primary structure (amino acid sequence) of the prion protein affects the physical structure, or 'three-dimensional shape', of the prion protein molecule, and the way in which it interacts with other biochemical events in the tissue.

What is the difference between PrP^c and PrP^{sc}?

This question brings us close to the core of the problem of prion disease. But as we move towards the central questions we arrive at the frontier of the understanding of prion disease. There are several theories about the mechanisms underlying the development of prion disease (the pathogenesis) and how prion disease might be transmitted, but proving which of these is correct is a matter of further experimentation and interpretation. It is generally accepted that PrP^c production is a normal cellular process that occurs throughout life in neurones and, to a lesser extent, in many other cell types in the body, and that PrP^c has an important normal, but unknown, function. Following the transcription of the genetic information from the gene into the RNA message and the translation of the RNA message into the basic amino acid sequence, the protein produced may be further modified. This *post-translational* modification may include the addition of non-amino acid components to the protein structure. For example, the prion protein molecule, PrP^c, has two amino acids that are capable of attaching large carbohydrate side-chains, both of which are occupied in most molecules. In addition, each PrP^c molecule has attached at its end a lipid-based component that anchors the molecule to the cell membrane of the cell in which it is synthesized. Newly synthesized protein will also take up a certain 'secondary structure', comprising the coils and loops in the string of amino acids, before folding up into the 'tertiary structure', its final three-dimensional shape. Changing from one structure to another requires energy and may be irreversible. When an egg is cooked the protein of the white of the egg absorbs energy and changes from a clear, colourless, runny substance to a white, opaque, rubbery substance. When the egg goes cold the white does not revert to its original state. In prion disease, the PrP^c molecules undergo a 'post-translational' change in state which seems to be irreversible. The nature of this change is not fully understood but it appears that PrP^c has a secondary structure in which the string of amino acids exists as several tightly wound coils, known as α-helices. This affects the way the protein then curls up into its final shape. The PrP^{sc} molecule has less α-helix content; rather, parts of the amino acid string line up next to each other to form a flat sheet, known as a β-pleated sheet. This means that the final shape of PrP^{sc} molecules is very different from that of PrP^c molecules. Proteins with a high β-pleated sheet content are very tough, which probably explains why PrP^{sc} is resistant to digestion with proteinase K. While this enzyme can get into the normal PrP^c molecule and digest it away completely, it can only manage to reduce PrP^{sc} to a protease-resistant core, PrP27–30. This core has a structure that encourages molecules to aggregate (a bit like Lego bricks) to form fibrils, which are recognized as amyloid in the brain. Both PrP^c and PrP^{sc} molecules have the same primary amino acid sequence and, so far, no real differences in post-translational processing, leading to changes in shape, have been uncovered, although it is accepted that the conversion of PrP^c to PrP^{sc} is a post-translational process. This conversion lies at the heart of Prusiner's prion hypothesis.

6

In the genes

A preliminary look at genes and proteins

Once a gene has been located and identified, methods are available for determining its sequence, that is, the order of 'bits of information' along the gene that ensures that the protein has all the appropriate amino acids (the building blocks of proteins) in the right order (the primary sequence, or primary structure). Each amino acid in the protein is coded for by one 'codon' or 'word' in the gene and each codon itself consists of three 'bases' or 'letters'. In the language of the genetic code, four different 'bases' are available, which are designated A, G, C, and T (from adenine, guanine, cytosine, and thymine). Thus, a nucleic acid consisting of a string of nine bases, for example, C–C–T–C–A–T–G–G–A, could potentially code for a protein, three amino acids long, with CCT coding for the first amino acid (in fact, an amino acid called proline), CAT for the second (histidine), and GGA for the third (glycine). There are, of course, 64 different three-letter words that can be produced from the four letters of the nucleic acid alphabet. There are, however, only about 20 different amino acids, so it is clear that there is some 'redundancy' in the relationship between nucleic acid code and amino acids, with some amino acids being encoded by more than one codon. For example, GGG, GGA, and GGT all code for glycine. There are also some three-letter words that do not code for an amino acid but which act as punctuations, signalling the end (or the start) of proteins. In addition to the sequences of bases determining the primary structure of the protein and those that determine the beginning and end of each protein, each gene also has long sequences of bases that do not code for the primary structure of the protein but which have other functions, though this will not be discussed further. Minor variations (known as mutations) in the base sequence will produce proteins having one or a few alterations in the amino acid sequence, but in most cases such a protein will still do its job more or less properly. During the course of protein manufacture, the information determining the amino acid sequence, encoded in the DNA (deoxyribonucleic acid) sequence of the gene is transcribed into a usable template in the form of RNA (ribonucleic acid). RNA also uses a four-base alphabet, with each DNA letter corresponding to a different RNA letter, so during transcription the order of letters in the DNA of the gene is faithfully reflected in the order of letters in the RNA. This messenger RNA carries its message from the nucleus (where the DNA is situated) to the protein factory within the cell where it is translated into the amino acid sequence of the protein. How much protein is being produced can be determined by the amount of messenger RNA specific to that protein.

Back to the PrP gene

By the mid-1980s it was known that human prion protein (PrP) consisted of a sequence of 254 amino acids and that the gene determining that sequence was located on chromosome 20. It was also known that prion protein occurred in all mammalian species with little variation in primary structure. For example, in mice the protein is 253 amino acids long and the gene is on mouse chromosome 2. Soon after the gene for PrP was identified, scientists found that in mice infected with scrapie agent the amount of PrP messenger RNA did not differ from that seen in normal animals. Evidence accumulated rapidly that the prion protein was a normal host protein doing a normal job most of the time but that it somehow 'went wrong' after it had been made (i.e. post-translation), and that this change was at the centre of the disease process.

As a result of genetic diversity, essentially the same protein will be slightly different in different species and in different individuals. It was immediately clear that variation in the prion protein gene (which we will call the PrP gene) was likely to be very important in determining differences in the way prion disease behaved in different animals or people. Nowhere was this more likely to be the case than in familial human prion disease and, although basic understanding of the mechanisms of prion disease progressed mainly in rodents, we will deal with the impact of molecular genetics on human disease first, since this elucidates many of the most important points.

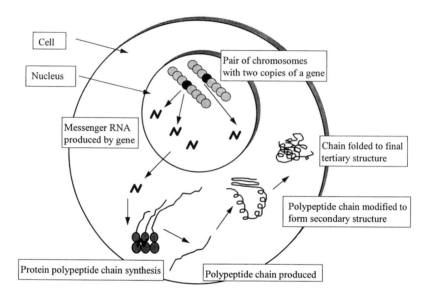

Cell

Nucleus

Pair of chromosomes
with two copies of a gene

Messenger RNA
produced by gene

Chain folded to final
tertiary structure

Polypeptide chain modified to
form secondary structure

Protein polypeptide chain synthesis

Polypeptide chain produced

Fig. 6.1 Simplified account of protein synthesis. Each cell (excluding sex cells) carries two copies of each gene, one inherited from each parent. The genes are arranged on pairs of chromosomes within the cell's nucleus and each cell contains 22 pairs of non-sex chromosomes (autosomes) and either two X chromosomes (females) or one X and one Y chromosome (males). One pair of chromosomes is shown and the two copies of a particular gene are shown, one on each chromosome. In many cases the two copies will be identical, but there is some variation in normal genes (alleles). As we have already described, there are two common alleles of the PrP gene, one encoding methionine at codon 129 and the other encoding valine at codon 129. So in our diagram the two highlighted gene copies could, for example, be PrP genes with both encoding methionine or valine, or with one encoding methionine and the other valine. The DNA sequence of both copies of the gene is transcribed into molecules of messenger RNA (mRNA) whose base sequence complements that of the gene. The mRNA molecules travel to the outer compartment of the cell where they act as templates for the synthesis of protein polypeptide chains (comprising strings of amino acids), the sequence of which is determined by the base sequence of the mRNA. Thus the primary sequence of the polypeptide chain is determined by the base sequence of the gene via the complementary mRNA. After the newly synthesized polypeptide chain is released from the synthetic mechanism, it is further modified chemically, for example, by the addition of side-chains, and folds into coils and sheets (secondary structure). The protein then folds up on itself to give the final three-dimensional (tertiary) structure. The amount of protein synthesis can be estimated by measuring the levels of mRNA within the tissue of interest.

The search for the cause of familial disease

In the mid-1980s, Prusiner had become aware of a Californian patient with GSS. Although this patient came from a family in which there had been a number of cases of a similar disease, he was the only family member who was ill at that time. Karen Hsiao with others in Prusiner's laboratory worked out the gene sequence for the PrP genes in this patient and in a large number of normal individual volunteers, and discovered that the patient had a mutation at codon number 102 in one copy of the PrP gene. In fact, he produced PrP which had the amino acid, leucine, at position 102, rather than the usual amino acid, proline. (Since everybody has two sets of chromosomes and, therefore, two copies of each gene, this patient actually produced equal amounts of two prion proteins, one with leucine and one with proline at position 102.) The question was whether this mutation accounted for this patient's illness or whether it was just a bit of the random variation in the protein that is frequently found between members of the same species, although the latter seemed unlikely since none of the normal volunteers encoded leucine at codon 102 of their PrP genes. This kind of question can often be resolved by analysing the gene in many people with a disease, and seeing whether the same mutation always occurs in people with the disease and not in those people who are not at risk of developing the disease. With a disease as rare as GSS there may be no more than a handful of people with the disease at any one time in the whole world. There was, however, frozen tissue stored from two members of the 'W' family described in Chapter 4. There were also several older members of that family who had outlived the usual age at onset for GSS, and who could be asked to donate blood. These people are particularly important because, in order to show that the disease is associated with one mutation, it is necessary to show that the disease is found in those people who do have the mutation but not in those older people from the same family who do not have the mutation. Additionally, there were many younger members of the family who were at 50 per cent risk of developing the illness, and many of these were asked to donate a blood sample for future research. Most of these people lived in southern England but a few lived in other parts of the world. Some lived in the United States and had to be contacted directly by Prusiner's laboratory. We and our colleagues collected blood from the UK members of the family. The blood samples were assembled in London and San Francisco and the analysis of the PrP genes was then undertaken. Not only did the original patient in California carry the mutation at codon 102 of the PrP gene, but tissue from the two deceased family members in Britain also carried the mutation. None of those family members who had outlived the risk period carried the mutation (Hsiao *et al.* 1989). This showed that the mutation and the disease were 'linked'. When assessing the degree of certainty with which it can be claimed that a gene mutation and a disease are linked, molecular geneticists calculate a probability figure known as the LOD score. In this family the LOD score was 3.2. A LOD score in excess of 3 means that the odds against the mutation and the disease being linked are less than 1 in 1000, and are sufficient to be reasonably certain that an individual who carried that mutation would develop disease.

This work was published in 1989, and GSS became the first neurological disease for which it was possible to name the exact gene mutation which would lead to illness. As we said earlier, there are perfectly normal variations in the base sequence of genes, which means that the proteins produced by these genes vary in different individuals, but they all do the job required. These common variations are called polymorphisms. By 1984, it was possible, using less precise techniques, to predict whether an at-risk individual would develop Huntington's disease, provided that a DNA sample was also available from a family member who was already ill, by comparing polymorphisms near to where the Huntington's gene was thought to be. In the case of GSS it was now possible to look right inside the relevant gene and to determine with great certainty whether the individual would develop the disease, even if there were no affected relatives available for comparison.

Looking into the future

What did this mean for the family who had donated the blood? Members of the 'W' family had known for a long time that they were at risk of inheriting a fatal disease and they knew that if one of their parents had the disease, they were at 50 per cent risk of developing disease themselves. The identification of the specific mutation meant that any member of the family could now find out with certainty whether or not they would develop the family disease. However, experience with families with Huntington's disease and some other adult-onset, fatal diseases suggested that this was unlikely to be a straightforward process. If family members decided that they did want to know whether or not they were carrying the mutant gene, they would have to go through the somewhat lengthy procedure of counselling, and then donate more blood. We do not know how the 'W' family reacted to these developments, or how many members underwent genetic testing, because we and our colleagues had been involved with the family in a *research* capacity; this was now a *clinical* matter in which it was not appropriate for us to be involved. There are, however, several studies on the complex issue of coping with a change from a 50 per cent risk to either a 0 per cent or, effectively, a 100 per cent risk of developing an adult-onset, fatal disease (Gray *et al.* 1996). The outcome of testing is likely to have important psychological effects for the person, their spouse or partner, and other family members, irrespective of whether it indicates an increased or decreased risk. There are also ethical problems. It is not appropriate to test a person without their informed consent, or if they are under 18 years old, or to divulge the result to a third party. There are also legal issues since life insurance and mortgage status may change. Then there is the problem of what to do if a person requests presymptomatic testing, but appears to be exhibiting symptoms which they themselves do not seem to acknowledge. They may be ready to be told that they have an increased risk of becoming ill, but they may not be ready to be told that they are already ill. Counselling consists of educating the 'client' (the term used in the context of genetic counselling) as to the exact nature of the risk and the implications for other relatives, particularly the client's children, together with a discussion of how the client is going to react to either a bad or a good outcome. Some people feel that it is an invasion of their privacy to have to go through all this to be given a piece of information which they feel they have a right to know. Others may feel that, unless they convince the counsellor that they have no problems, they will not be told the answer. They may, therefore, conceal their anxieties and not benefit from the counselling that is offered. Without counselling a person may think they want to know what their risk is, only to find out afterwards that they wished they had not been told.

Being told that the test indicates that disease is certain, provided the patient is not carried off by something else, is very difficult to bear, although many clients who are given this news seem to cope reasonably well. Many will have lived with a 50 per cent risk for many years and may be approaching an age at which disease onset might be imminent. Some will have already noticed subtle changes in their behaviour, which they believe indicate the onset of the disease, so for them a test is almost a diagnosis. But the human mind is very subtle and can present unexpected difficulties. People who have coped well with the knowledge that they are living with a 50 per cent risk of illness may become very depressed on being told that disease is certain, and then feel deeply disappointed by their own inability to deal with something that they thought they could handle. They may feel guilty that they may have passed on the mutant gene to their children, because an increase in risk of illness from 50 per cent to 100 per cent in the parent raises the risk in offspring from 25 per cent to 50 per cent. The age at onset of familial prion disease varies between 30 and 70 years. So, even though these people know they will eventually become ill, they do not know exactly *when* and are, therefore, still left with an uncertain future. They may not become sick for many years and they are not protected from other serious illnesses, such as cancer, which may occur when they are in their 50s.

Clients whose tests indicate that they are not carrying the mutant gene and are not at risk of developing the disease may be pleased initially, but then go on to have complex psychological difficulties. This has sometimes been referred to as 'survivor guilt'. Many families afflicted with this sort of disease become very close-knit, as family members share the burden of a risk of illness. Genetic testing divides the family, and people who are no longer at risk may feel left out. People who find that they are no longer at risk actually feel guilty at having previously developed a self-image which turned out not to be based on fact, rather than recognizing that such an image was one way of coping with an awful problem. Many people have an imperfect grasp of the concept of chance and believe that, if their brother or sister is told that the risk of becoming ill is less than was thought, that increases their own risk, which, of course, it does not. Some people living with a 50 per cent risk may behave unambitiously, others may behave irresponsibly. When, after testing, they learn that they are not at risk of developing the disease they may regret their earlier behaviour. Being at 50 per cent risk may be used as an excuse for any sort of behaviour or personality trait, and can make a person feel in some way 'special'. Having this aspect of their self-image removed, by being told that they are not at risk, may be difficult to adjust to. Realizing that they had turned a 50 per cent risk into a kind of 'advantage' could be psychologically devastating. Layer upon layer of psychological adjustment may be needed before the client feels comfortable.

There are also many difficulties for the spouse or partner of a person who receives a change in risk status. In any relationship there is a complex pattern of support and dependency which inevitably changes with a change in risk. The divorce rate amongst couples, one of whom is told that their risk of illness is lower than was thought, is *higher* than amongst couples, one of whom is told that their risk of illness is increased. Couples who share the knowledge that one partner is at 50 per cent risk of developing a fatal disease in middle age, build the possibility that the partner might die prematurely into their relationship. If the at-risk partner is tested and is cleared of risk, he or she may become more assertive and less dependent on the other partner, who may feel ashamed to realize that he or she had been expecting to survive longer. All these adjustments take time, and counselling is usually taken at a fairly slow pace. Despite having spent half a lifetime wondering whether it was going to happen to them, the majority of people offered genetic counselling for fatal, adult-onset disorders choose not to be tested.

Looking into the womb

There is one situation, however, where presymptomatic testing does have specific implications. This is prenatal testing. In theory it is possible to test the early fetus and to terminate the pregnancy if the fetus carries the abnormal gene, thus ensuring that a person's children and all their future descendants will be free of the disease for ever. In practice the situation is rarely that simple. In many cases the diagnosis of a late-onset disorder is not made until a person's own children are young adults. Such a young adult may, therefore, be faced with dealing with a sick parent, the recent discovery of their own risk, and the imminent arrival of their own children. When a fetal test indicates the presence of the abnormal gene, the risk status of the parent is then immediately obvious. It is appropriate to test a fetus only when the decision to terminate a pregnancy in the event of an adverse outcome has already been taken. This is because it is impossible to maintain the child's right not to know their risk status later in life if a parent is given that information, since the parents are unlikely to be able to conceal it from the child, however hard they try. However, parents may have indicated that they plan a termination, only to find that they do not wish to go through with it later, by which time the risk status of the fetus may have been determined. The emotional trauma of the prospect of a late abortion can add greatly to the pressure under which couples may find themselves. In the UK, abortion is legal in the case of a serious genetic defect in the fetus, and familial prion disease would normally be considered to fall into this category because it usually has an age at onset in middle life. It is becoming increasingly difficult to know how to cope with the growing number of very late-onset disorders which can now be predicted. Many people feel that there are ethical problems in prenatal testing for diseases that are only going to become a problem very late in life. In practice, the occasions when prenatal testing for adult-onset illnesses is a positive option are very limited.

Looking into the past

Molecular genetic analysis is also a way of looking into the past. In 1986, we attempted transmission of spongiform encephalopathy to marmosets by intracerebral injection of brain tissue from a patient who had died of a rather unusual dementing illness in which there had been a mild form of spongiform encephalopathy. In the event, the transmission was unsuccessful, in that the monkeys survived for 5 years without signs of illness. This was interesting in view of other evidence to show that this patient undoubtedly died of a prion disease. Molecular analysis of his PrP gene showed that it contained a small additional piece of DNA (Owen *et al.* 1989). In the normal prion protein, which is 254 amino acids long, there is a section between amino acids 50 and 90 (that is, 40 amino acids long) in which a sequence of eight amino acids (an octapeptide) is repeated, with minor differences, five times. This patient had an extra six repetitions, making 11 repetitions in all. The section of the PrP gene encoding the normal amino acid repeat sequence is 120 bases long (5 repeats × 8 codons × 3 bases per codon = 120 bases). This extra repeat sequence contained 144 bases (actually pairs of bases—see the glossary for an explanation of base pairs) and is therefore referred to as the 144 bp repeat sequence. This abnormality was found shortly before the codon 102 mutation described in the previous sections but, because tissue was available from only one affected person, it was not possible to be sure whether these extra repeat sequences were responsible for the illness or whether their presence was merely coincidental. In other words, our colleagues had not been able to calculate a LOD score.

Enquiries of family members indicated that the patient's father, George, had died of a neurological illness nearly 40 years earlier and had, in fact, been the first described case of the so-called Heidenhain variant of CJD, published in a report in 1954 (Meyer *et al.* 1954). According to the report of 1954, George had no other affected relatives, but the fact that his son had now died and had a heritable abnormality in his PrP gene made it likely that the abnormality was responsible for the disease in both father and son. The problem was to prove it. When we and our colleagues discussed these cases with neurologists and neuropathologists, mainly in the London area, they told us that they knew other patients with a very similar disease, who were either alive or who had died recently, and from whom blood or other tissue samples were available. Our colleagues found that 11 of these cases were harbouring the same 144 bp insertion within their PrP genes. This made it undoubtedly true that the gene abnormality was responsible for their illness. However, these 11 people came from four apparently unconnected families. Mutations occur spontaneously as errors in the copying of DNA and will be inherited by a proportion of the descendants, provided, of course, that the mutant protein is not incompatible with survival of the offspring and does not compromise reproductive capacity. But spontaneous mutation is an extremely rare event and it seemed unlikely that these 144 bp insertion cases were unrelated.

Enquiries from the patients' relatives quickly established that two of the families were related, but proving that this group was related to the other two families required a great deal of detective work. Two of our colleagues, Mark Poulter and Ray Lofthouse, spent much of the summer of 1990 working their way through data available at the Registry General of Births, Deaths and Marriages at St Catherine's House, London. By searching the Marriage Index, Ray and Mark were able to identify the occupation and place of residence of the parents of each patient, and the mother's maiden name.

By searching the Death Register covering the years in which the parents might have died, they were able to infer which parent was more likely to have been affected by the family disease. Death certificates detail the cause and the place of death, although the recorded cause of death is often unhelpful. It may, for example, just specify pneumonia without indicating what else was wrong with the patient. However, the place of death was often either a psychiatric hospital, a nursing home, or geriatric hospital and, if the patient died while still in middle age, our colleagues usually proceeded on the assumption that this person (rather than the spouse) had died of the disease, and went in search of their parents.

In addition to working backwards through the generations in this way, it was also necessary for Ray and Mark to come back down the generations, in order to find the links to the other affected patients who carried the same mutation. By working through the register of births for the years on either side of the birth of a particular case, it was often possible to identify their brothers and sisters. By working up from other affected patients it would then become apparent that their parents or grandparents were the brothers or sisters of people whose descendants were part of the other families. In this way the families were joined up, and many other branches which also suffered from the disease were discovered.

This laborious process involved waiting several days at each stage as the

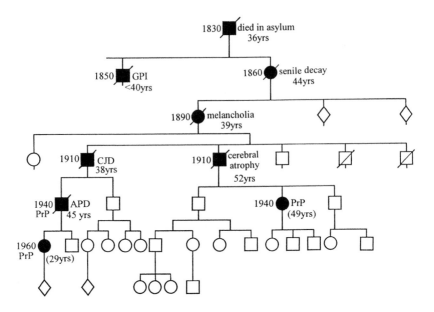

Fig. 6.2 Part of a pedigree of a family in which prion disease is inherited in an autosomal dominant pattern, that is, one in which about half of the offspring of a person who subsequently becomes affected will themselves eventually be affected. Squares indicate males; circles indicate females; diamonds indicate people of unknown gender. Filled symbols indicate affected members. Dates show the decade of birth. Age is age at death (except for those in brackets where age is age at onset in patients alive at the time the tree was prepared). Death certificates and hospital notes were used to assess the diagnosis. The patient at the top of the tree could be identified only as having died in an asylum at a young age. His elder son was diagnosed as suffering from GPI, general paralysis of the insane, an old name for neurosyphilis, which may be a misdiagnosis. The daughter died of 'senile decay' which we can take to mean dementia. In the next generation, one woman died from 'melancholia' in an asylum. This usually means depression, but a dementing illness could have received this diagnosis. Two of her five sons died from a brain disease in middle age. The daughter of the younger of these sons became ill at the end of the 1980s. DNA analysis showed that she carried the 144 bp insertion in her PrP gene. The other son had a neuropathological examination post-mortem, and a diagnosis of CJD was made. His son later became ill and neuropathological examination of the brain indicated that he had a prion disease of an unusual nature, but the detection of the 144 bp insertion confirmed the diagnosis of atypical prion disease. When his daughter developed neurological symptoms, DNA analysis showed that she also carried the 144 bp insertion. Where distant cousins carry the same mutation, all the intervening ancestors that link the two cousins are obligate carriers, that is, they must also carry the mutation.

certificates were copied and made ready for collection. It also involved deeply frustrating hold-ups because, for common names, there might be more than one person who could have been part of a family, and it was only when the certificates came through that the correct people could be identified. Sometimes the trail went cold because both parents died young, or illegitimacy prevented the father from being identified. The method worked as far back as 1831 when the national registration of births, deaths, and marriages in Great Britain began. Mark and Ray found that all the affected people whose gene had been tested came from four families resident in three villages in Sussex at the beginning of the nineteenth century. After consulting the parish records kept in the churches of these three villages, and the 10-yearly census records kept at the Public Record Office in London, they discovered that the four ancestors were all brothers and sisters of each other, and that all those people who carried a 144 bp insertion within the PrP gene were descended from a Sussex couple who lived at the end of the eighteenth century. Of course the mutation may have occurred much further back in time than that, but our colleagues did not pursue their search.

Having built up the extended family tree and decided which of the family members were carrying the mutant gene, we were able to look back at the diagnoses as recorded on the death certificates and, in many cases, the hospital records obtained from the hospitals in which these people had died. We were therefore able to see what prion disease had looked like before it was recognized as a specific disease (Collinge *et al.* 1992; Poulter *et al.* 1992). The age at onset ranged from 28 to 53 years, men and women were equally likely to be affected, and on average half of each sibship (set of brothers and sisters) were affected. One parent was either clearly, or very probably, affected in each family. In other words, the pattern of disease was consistent with dominant inheritance. All patients showed a progressive dementia, with a variety of motor symptoms being seen in some patients. In some cases, the neurological illness was preceded by personality changes, psychiatric disorders such as depression, or antisocial and aggressive behaviour. Sometimes the antisocial behaviour preceded the onset of clinical symptoms by many years. The duration of illness ranged from 1 to 18 years, although the majority of patients were ill for 4–7 years. Brain pathology could only be examined in four cases and these showed changes which had a somewhat unusual form of spongiform encephalopathy. This, together with the long duration of illness, made it appropriate to give these patients a modern diagnosis of 'atypical prion disease'. Diagnoses up to the Second World War had tended to be either correct but non-specific, such as, 'brain disease', 'decay of dementia', 'exhaustion from dementia', and 'cerebral softening'. There was also the somewhat quaint 'dementia due to religion'. Now what could that have meant? In later years the diagnoses became more specific but not necessarily accurate, for example, Alzheimer's disease (the most common form of dementia in old age, which can occasionally have a onset in middle age), Huntington's disease (the best known hereditary neurodegenerative disease), or Pick's disease (a rare form of dementia with severe personality changes). The first 'correct' diagnosis of Heidenhain's syndrome was made in 1948, followed by a diagnosis of CJD in 1950 in a distant cousin.

It was possible to identify 'obligate carriers' within the extended pedigree. These are people who, because of their position in a family tree, must have carried the mutation. For example, where two first cousins are affected then the parent of one, who is also the aunt or uncle of the other, must also have carried the gene. Some of these obligate carriers died in early middle age in circumstances which suggested that they may have been suffering from the family disease even though this was not directly the cause of death. Such causes of death included suicide, bronchopneumonia, bedsores (indicating that the person had been bedridden for a long time), and fatal accidents. Several patients in this family were described as having died of 'general paralysis of the insane', which means the terminal dementia of the venereal

Table 6.1 Historical diagnoses in a pedigree with inherited prion disease

Year	Diagnosis	Year	Diagnosis
1864	Decay of dementia	1950	Huntington's disease; CJD
1868	General paralysis of the insane	1961	Presenile atrophy
1885	Brain disease	1964	Presenile dementia; Parkinson's disease
1891	Decay of epilepsy	1966	Presenile dementia
1894	General paralysis of the insane	1968	Pick's disease (two cases)
1895	Dementia due to religion	1974	Presenile dementia (two cases)
1901	General paralysis of the insane	1983	Myoclonic epilepsy
1910	Dementia solicited by lactation	1986	Huntington's disease
1912	Senile decay	1986	Huntington's disease
1923	General paralysis of the insane	1987	Huntington's disease and/or Alzheimer's disease
1930	Dementia praecox (schizophrenia)		
1930	Cerebral thrombosis	1987	Alzheimer's disease
1933	Exhaustion due to dementia	1989	Alzheimer's disease
1937	Cerebral softening	1990	Huntington's disease and/or Alzheimer's disease
1946	Epilepsy and dementia		

disease, syphilis. This was probably a misdiagnosis, although it is possible that they also had syphilis. The limited medical notes that could be obtained were not inconsistent with prion disease, and the age of death was certainly appropriate. The LOD score for this family was calculated to be more than 11 which meant that the odds that the 144 bp insertion in the PrP gene and the disease were not linked were less than 1 in 10^{11} (one hundred thousand million).

More mutations

Following the discovery of these two mutations in the PrP gene in two families with human prion disease, other mutations within the gene were soon found in other families. There are likely to be in excess of 30 mutations within this gene which can lead to familial prion disease, each with a slightly different but overlapping clinical picture. It had been quite fortuitous that the patient in California and the 'W' family in Britain had shared the same mutation, because, if they had had different mutations within the same gene, linkage to disease would have been more difficult to establish. There is no reason to suppose that the Californian patient was even remotely related to the 'W' family, and there are some other genetic reasons to suggest that he was not. This mutation (designated Pro102Leu, and indicating a proline to leucine change in amino acid at codon 102) has now been found in Japanese patients, which indicates, almost certainly, that it has occurred spontaneously on separate occasions. Affected descendants of the first GSS case to be described, back in the 1930s, have been shown to carry the Pro102Leu mutation, indicating that the disease now described as GSS and that reported by Gerstmann, Sträussler and Scheinker are one and the same (Kretzchmar *et al.* 1991).

Several unresolved puzzles were also solved by the new techniques of molecular genetic analysis. For example, all the cases of CJD amongst the Libyan Jews were found to carry a mutation at codon 200 of the PrP gene (Glu200Lys, involving an amino acid change from glutamate to lysine at codon 200), proving that the high incidence of CJD within this ethnic group was familial rather than caused by eating sheep's brain or eyeballs, as had been originally suggested. Similar clusters of CJD in Slovakia, Chile, and various other parts of the world were found to be associated with this Glu200Lys mutation, which now accounts for the majority of cases of familial CJD. The clinical picture in these cases is indistinguishable from that of the more common, sporadic cases of CJD.

Another mutation, causing a disease similar to familial CJD in a large family in France, was found at codon 178 (Asp178Asn, involving an amino acid change from aspartic acid to asparagine at codon 178). Subsequently, by extracting DNA from fixed tissue scraped off microscope slides, which had been stored for more than 50 years, scientists were able to show that the familial cases first described by Jakob had also carried the codon 178 mutation (Brown *et al.* 1994). Rather special techniques are required in order to extract usable DNA from completely dead tissue. The extraction of intact DNA from the preserved remains of mammoths and dinosaurs, as portrayed in the movie *Jurassic Park*, may be unrealistic as yet, but such techniques are becoming very important in forensic investigations and in some branches of archaeology.

The large pedigree from Indiana, which has a unique neuropathological picture reminiscent of both prion disease and Alzheimer's disease, has a mutation at codon 198 of the PrP gene (Phe198Ser, involving an amino acid change from phenylalanine to serine at codon 198). As far as we know, this mutation has not been found in any other family. This pedigree, known in the literature as the Indiana kindred, and some other cases in which the neuropathology shares some of the features of both Alzheimer's disease and prion disease, suggest that prion disease should not be regarded as so categorically different from other neurodegenerative diseases, as the demonstration of the transmissibility of prion disease had at first suggested. In other words, what emerged as a distinct disease entity in the 1970s and 1980s is now beginning to look more like one end of a spectrum of diseases which are linked by the involvement of various unusual features of protein metabolism.

A number of families have been found which have abnormal repeat sequences in the PrP gene. As we discussed above, the normal PrP gene has five repeats of an eight amino acid sequence between codons 50 and 90. The large UK pedigree with an extra six repeats was the first with an insertion mutation to be reported. Families with an extra one, two, four, five, seven, eight, or nine repeats have now been described, and most of these insertions are associated with severe neurological disease. This part of the PrP gene may, therefore, be rather unstable and prone to copying errors. Some individuals from the general population are occasionally found to carry variations in the octapeptide repeat sequence which are not associated with disease. This finding illustrates how important it is not to rely totally on genetic analysis in diagnosis. If the PrP gene of people with any mild, neurological symptoms is analysed, and found to contain previously unknown mutations, it cannot be assumed that that person has prion disease. Only when enough patients with that mutation have been found to demonstrate a statistically significant association between illness and the mutation can genetic analysis be used as a diagnostic tool. Even then it is important to establish, by careful clinical diagnosis, that a person who carries one of these mutations is really developing prion disease. There is a risk that a patient, who is known to be carrying a PrP mutation, may be denied treatment for another, treatable illness if their symptoms are too rapidly attributed to the onset of prion disease.

It had always been difficult to diagnose cases of familial prion disease. However, the dual developments of PrP antibody staining of the brain and the identification of mutations in the PrP gene made the demarcation between prion diseases and other dementing conditions much more clear-cut, and helped to identify cases which would otherwise have been missed. The identification of more than 20 mutations within the PrP gene leading to familial prion disease helped to subdivide the familial diseases. Familial cases with a codon 200 mutation had a disease whose symptoms and neuropathology were indistinguishable from sporadic CJD, while the remaining mutations tended to produce a longer disease duration and the deposition of various forms of plaques and other PrP deposits in the brain. But this was not invariably the case. In the 'W' family referred to above, one person had a disease indistinguishable from CJD, one person became the definitive clinical description of GSS, several other family members resembled this case to a remarkable degree, while at least two members of the family had a disease which, although undoubtedly a prion disease, could only be described as 'atypical'. One day the reason for these differences may become clear, but they probably lie within the genetic make-up of the affected person.

The PrP gene in all of us

Genetic mutations arise when errors are made in the copying of DNA when new cells are made. If mutations occur in egg or sperm cells, they pass down through all subsequent generations. Mutations that have harmful effects do not spread widely throughout populations because, on average, people who suffer from those effects have fewer children. Many mutations are harmless or even beneficial and these can spread widely throughout a species. These common variations in a gene are called polymorphisms, and an important polymorphism is found in the PrP gene at codon 129. This codon produces either the amino acid valine or methionine at this position in the prion protein. Amongst Caucasians (Whites) about 38 per cent of people carry two copies of the methionine-encoding gene and 11 per cent carry two copies of the valine-encoding gene. These people are described as being MM or VV homozygous, respectively. The remaining 51 per cent of this population carries one copy of each gene and are described as MV heterozygous. Racial groups differ in the proportions of these three types. For example, most Japanese are MM homozygous.

In a *Lancet* paper in 1991, John Collinge and his colleagues at St Mary's hospital in London reported their gene analysis of the first few human growth hormone CJD cases, most of which were VV129 homozygous, the least common genotype found in the European population (Collinge *et al.* 1991). This might have suggested that VV129 homozygotes were very susceptible to developing CJD if treated with contaminated growth hormone and that the other two genotypes were unsusceptible. As more cases came to light, however, it became clear that both VV129 and MM129 homozygotes were susceptible and that some 90 per cent of all iatrogenic cases were homozygous at codon 129, compared with about 50 per cent of the general population. The Collinge team also reported that codon 129 is of importance, not only in the iatrogenic cases of CJD, but also in the sporadic cases (Palmer *et al.* 1991).

Variations on a theme

As we analysed the data from the UK family with the 144 bp insertion, we noticed that the ages at onset fell into two groups; 'young onset', where the patient became ill at 35–47 years of age, and 'late onset', where age at onset was between 53 and 65 years. Did this polymorphism, which affected the structure of the PrP protein, also affect the course of the disease in people who carried another mutation in that gene, and who were therefore destined to become sick? The 144 bp mutation occurred in a PrP gene that coded for methionine at codon 129 in all members of this family. This relationship was not likely to change since the whole gene would be inherited from one parent. What about the other PrP gene which had been inherited from the other parent (who from the perspective of this disease had married in) and would vary between people in different parts of the pedigree? Genetic testing indicated that those people who carried methionine on the other PrP gene belonged to the early onset age group, and those that carried valine belonged to the late-onset age group. Thus, a common variation in the PrP gene, which is found in all the population, was influencing the course of this very rare disease. It turned out that what mattered most was not that the other PrP gene carried a methionine but that it carried the same amino acid at codon 129 as the mutated gene carried. This homozygosity at codon 129 was to become very important in understanding other forms of prion disease. Although the PrP gene holds the key to many features of prion disease, other genes clearly also make a contribution. The clinical picture and neuropathology seen in Chinese and Japanese patients is frequently different from that seen in Caucasian patients. Even within families where the mutant genes are identical there is considerable variation in disease presentation between patients.

The special relationship of FFI and CJD

The genetic basis of the form of prion disease known as FFI (fatal familial insomnia) is particularly subtle. Patients with this form of disease were found to carry a mutation at codon 178 of the PrP gene. So were people from other families (including Jakob's first familial cases) who had 'classical' CJD. What was going on? The patients from families with FFI were found to encode methionine at codon 129 of the mutated PrP gene, while patients from families with CJD were found to encode a valine at codon 129 of the mutated gene. This variation did not just produce different symptoms. The neuropathology in FFI was very different from that seen in CJD. It was confined largely to the subcortical areas of the brain. So, just one amino acid change at position 129 of the PrP gene could change the disease, the occurrence of which was determined by the amino acid at position 178 of the PrP gene, from one form of prion disease into another (Goldfarb *et al.* 1992). It has recently been found that patients with the Pro102Leu mutation who carry valine at codon 129 on the same copy of the PrP gene have a very different clinical and pathological picture than patients with Pro102Leu mutation and methionine at codon 129.

There was a final twist to the story. The amino acid at codon 129 of the *other* PrP gene also made a contribution. Those patients with either FFI or CJD who had the same amino acid at position 129 of both PrP proteins had an earlier age at onset and more rapidly progressive disease than those who carried one of each amino acid. In this respect they resemble members of the 144 bp family described above. These results illustrate the exquisite sensitivity of the disease to the precise genetic defect, irrespective of lifestyle. In 1979, long before any of these mutations had been identified, Paul

Brown, who had spent many years collating data on the occurrence of CJD, was prompted to ask whether 'all the cards have already been dealt before a patient is born?' (Brown and Cathala 1979).

Genes and plaques

As the geneticists began to talk to the neuropathologists about these interesting developments, further patterns in these diseases emerged. Sporadic cases of CJD who had PrP plaques in the brain (about 10 per cent of the total) were found to carry at least one valine at codon 129 of the PrP gene, whereas the remainder (who were methionine homozygous at codon 129) did not have plaques (MacDonald *et al.* 1996). However, those iatrogenic cases of CJD who developed disease following intramuscular injections of contaminated growth hormone, *all* had PrP plaques, irrespective of what they carried at codon 129 (Ironside 1996*b*). This suggested either that there was something special about the PrP^{sc} which contaminated the growth hormone, or that there was something about acquisition of the disease from an external source via a peripheral (non-brain) route of infection that was causing people who were methionine homozygotes to produce plaques. The majority of people with kuru also had plaques in their brains. A recent analysis of stored material from kuru victims and unaffected people from Papua New Guinea shows that, although valine at codon 129 was slightly more common in this ethnic group than in Westerners, there was no difference in the PrP genotypes between people with and without kuru (Hainfellner *et al.* 1997). This suggests, first, that people who are heterozygous at codon 129 are not protected from kuru in the same way as they appear to be protected from sporadic or iatrogenic CJD. Secondly, although a detailed analysis of the relationship between codon 129 and PrP plaques in kuru has yet to be undertaken, the raw data suggest that people with kuru who are homozygous for methionine at codon 129 can have PrP plaques in their brains. This relationship between the PrP gene and the occurrence of PrP plaques in the brain turned out to be an important factor in identifying the new variant of CJD, which may be caused by BSE. This shows how careful and methodical work can have an important 'pay-off' many years later. When the new variant of CJD was identified in Britain in 1996, all the early cases were homozygous for methionine at codon 129 and all had PrP plaques, albeit of rather unusual shapes. This made the new variant cases more like acquired cases than sporadic cases and, in addition to their young age, was a good indicator that something new was occurring. Conversely, this analysis added weight to the view that sporadic cases were not acquired from an external source. However, while this view is accepted by most workers in the field, there are still some who feel that 'every case of CJD must have been caught from somewhere'.

7

Transgenes, transplants, and test tubes

In 1982, Stan Prusiner had published a long paper in the prestigious journal, *Science*, entitled 'Novel proteinaceous infectious particles cause scrapie'. In this paper he reviewed a series of experiments carried out either in his own laboratory or by other groups and in earlier times, which confirm that the scrapie agent is not inactivated by techniques that specifically destroy nucleic acid, such as irradiation, high temperatures, or treatment with enzymes. He also provided evidence that techniques capable of destroying proteins, especially enzymes that break up proteins, markedly reduced infectivity. These data, together with the very small size of the scrapie agent, led Prusiner to suggest that the scrapie agent consisted of either '(i) a small nucleic acid surrounded by a tightly packed protein coat or (ii) a protein devoid of nucleic acid, that is, an infectious protein'.

If in the first of these suggestions he means a nucleic acid too small to code for a protein structure, then he is referring to something like a 'virino'. The second of these suggestions, as stated, and on Prusiner's admission, is heretical. However, Prusiner then went on to explore various ways in which an agent consisting only of protein, which he called a 'prion', might be infectious. ('Prion' is derived from *pro*teinaceous *in*fectious. It should, logically, have been called a 'proin', but somehow that does not trip off the tongue so well! By using the word prion as a noun rather than an adjective, Prusiner seemed to be emphasizing that the prion protein was behaving like a micro-organism, different from but comparable to a virus, rather than like other proteins, which are merely very complex chemicals. Many scientists found this difficult to swallow, and while the term 'prion protein' has gained universal currency, many in the field, including ourselves, prefer to avoid the use of 'prions'.) One of Prusiner's suggestions was that prion protein might activate a host gene to produce more prion protein. This begs the question of why the host should carry such a potentially disadvantageous gene, leading to the further suggestion that the gene might also code for some other essential protein. This essential protein would be sufficiently similar to the prion protein that the two would be immunologically indistinguishable. This would explain why the host did not 'notice' the infection. It may be asked how one gene could make two, albeit related, proteins, since the codon sequence in the gene determines the amino acid sequence in the protein. This is a problem but, in fact, protein molecules are subject to a great deal of processing both during synthesis and after they have been formed, so that different versions of the same protein can be manufactured from one gene. This was the nearest that Prusiner's 1982 paper came to what is now accepted to be the relationship between the PrP gene and the infectious agent, but much more work was required before this became clear.

The 1990s: the ascendance of prion protein

The value of a scientific theory is judged by the simplicity of its explanations for real events, as well as its power to predict events which can then be substantiated or refuted by experiments. One of the most elegant aspects of the notion that the infectious agent of prion disease is a modified form of a host-coded protein is that it begins to make sense of the familial, sporadic, and acquired patterns of occurrence of human (and to some extent animal) prion disease in the natural world. The observation that in familial human prion disease, an apparently genetic defect gives rise to an illness which can then be experimentally transmitted to animals, becomes a possibility, although it remains an astonishing phenomenon. As we saw in the last chapter these familial prion diseases are associated with mutations in the PrP gene. These mutant genes will produce prion protein with slightly different amino acid sequences and, therefore, slightly different secondary and tertiary structures. The different structures will alter the stability of the three-dimensional shape of the molecule, and alter the probability with which it can undergo a spontaneous change in shape, including the irreversible change from PrP^c to PrP^{sc}. A high probability that this process will be initiated by middle age in people who carry certain mutations in the PrP gene explains why these people inevitably become ill as they get older. For some of the mutations in the PrP gene, disease onset is not until later middle age or even old age. A proportion of the people who carry these mutations may escape the disease by dying of some other illness, but calculations which correct for death from other causes suggest that everyone who carries a pathogenic mutation in the PrP gene will develop prion disease if they live long enough. The general population carry what is called the 'wild-type' PrP gene, and the PrP^c molecules that it produces are very stable in that the probability that they will undergo spontaneous conversion to PrP^{sc} molecules is extremely low, but not zero. This accounts for the one in a million incidence of prion disease in the general population.

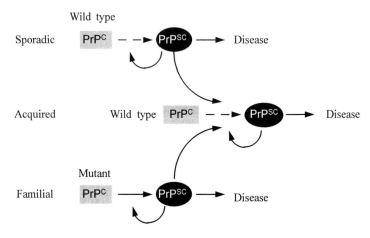

Fig. 7.1 The relationship between sporadic, acquired, and familial prion diseases in humans. In sporadic prion disease, the probability that PrP^c will convert to PrP^{sc} spontaneously is extremely low, but once the process has started it is autocatalytic (sustained by positive feedback) and disease will result. In acquired cases, the conversion of PrP^c to PrP^{sc} is initiated by PrP^{sc} from an outside source (by contamination), and sustained by positive feedback, leading to disease. In familial prion disease, a mutation in the PrP gene ensures that the PrP^c produced is more likely to convert to PrP^{sc} so that disease is inevitable by late middle age.

The twist in the story comes when one looks at acquired cases of prion disease. Since infectivity is related to the presence of PrP^{sc} in a tissue preparation, it appears that one factor that stimulates the conversion of PrP^c to PrP^{sc} is the presence of some PrP^{sc}. Thus, contamination with PrP^{sc} from an outside source can trigger the disease. For some years this has been a description of what appears to be the case, although little progress has been made in explaining what it is about PrP^{sc} that can stimulate the conversion of PrP^c to PrP^{sc}. The reader will note, however, that what the PrP^{sc} molecules are doing is converting the three-dimensional shape of existing PrP^c molecules into the PrP^{sc} shape, and that PrP^{sc} molecules are not strictly replicating themselves by manufacturing chemically new PrP^{sc} molecules.

The prion hypothesis

Prusiner's prion hypothesis argues that PrP^{sc} is itself the infectious agent in the spongiform encephalopathies. Although he often refers to prion *replication*, he does not mean it to be understood in the same way as virus replication. In the latter, virus infection of a cell leads to the synthesis of exact copies of the virus; in the case of prion replication, the infecting PrP^{sc} causes the host PrP^c to convert to the abnormal conformation (shape). The newly produced PrP^{sc} molecules need not be exact copies of the infecting PrP^{sc} which may actually have come from another species.

The prion hypothesis can be summarized briefly as follows. In individuals carrying the normal, wild-type PrP gene, the gene product, PrP^c, has a very low probability of spontaneously converting to the PrP^{sc} conformation by later middle age. This probability leads to the general incidence of sporadic CJD of about one per million of the population. In those families inheriting one of the pathogenic mutations in the PrP gene, the mutant PrP^c has a much higher probability of converting to PrP^{sc} by later middle age. For most mutations this probability will approach certainty, so that those family members carrying the mutant PrP gene are guaranteed to develop prion disease. According to the prion hypothesis, once molecules of PrP^{sc} are formed, each interacts with a normal PrP^c molecule to form a heterodimer (a double molecule) and, in this interaction, PrP^{sc} acts as a template to convert the PrP^c into PrP^{sc}. The heterodimer then dissociates into two PrP^{sc} molecules which can then form heterodimers with new PrP^c molecules. If brain tissue from an individual with prion disease, say a human, is injected into the brain of an animal, say a monkey, the infecting human PrP^{sc} interacts with the normal monkey PrP^c and converts it to monkey PrP^{sc}. This newly formed monkey PrP^{sc} will interact with more monkey PrP^c to set off a chain reaction, producing more and more monkey PrP^{sc} until the animal becomes ill. The infectious agent does not need an independent, information-carrying, nucleic acid genome. The key event is the PrP^{sc}-catalysed conversion of PrP^c to PrP$^{sc.}$ It might be supposed that the efficiency of this conversion will depend on the similarity in structure between the infecting PrP^{sc} and the host PrP^c, a similarity reflected by the similarity in primary sequence. There is considerable evidence that this is true. As mentioned above, the primary transmission of spongiform encephalopathy from one species to another (say from sheep to mouse) will involve a longer incubation time than subsequent serial transmissions from mouse to mouse. This species-barrier effect reflects the difference in primary sequence between sheep PrP^{sc} and mouse PrP^{c}. The primary sequences of mouse PrP^{sc} and mouse PrP^{c} are identical, so transmission between mice is more efficient, as shown by a shorter incubation period.

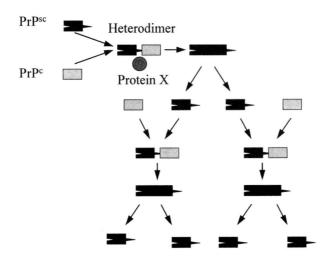

Fig. 7.2 Schematic illustrating the basic prion hypothesis, which says that molecules of PrP^{sc} will combine with molecules of PrP^{c} to form heterodimers (mixed pairs). During this interaction, the PrP^{c} will convert to PrP^{sc}. The two molecules of PrP^{sc} are then able to separate and to go in search of further PrP^{c} molecules. Studies using transgenic mice suggest that another molecule, designated protein X, may also be involved in the conversion process.

This is where the modern technique of transgenics begins to make a contribution. It is now possible to take the ovum (female reproductive cell or egg) from a mouse and add or subtract individual genes. The egg is then fertilized with sperm (male reproductive cells of which only one cell fertilizes the egg) and transplanted into the womb of an adult female mouse. When the offspring, known as a transgenic mouse, is born it has the characteristics determined by all its genes, including the ones which were added. That the species barrier is dependent on the degree of similarity (homology) between PrP molecules has been proved by studies using transgenic mice. David Westaway, working in Prusiner's laboratory, carried out some very elegant experiments in which transgenic mice were created which carried copies of the hamster PrP gene in addition to the normal mouse PrP gene (Westaway *et al.* 1992). Normal mice, when injected with hamster PrP^{sc} develop disease after a much longer incubation time than when they are injected with mouse PrP^{sc}. When transgenic mice carrying copies of the hamster PrP gene are injected with hamster PrP^{sc}, this difference in incubation time is abolished. Furthermore, when *mouse* PrP^{sc} is used to infect these transgenic mice, the accumulating PrP^{sc} is *mouse* PrP^{sc}. When *hamster* PrP^{sc} is used to infect these animals, the accumulating PrP^{sc} is *hamster* PrP^{sc}. In other words, the infecting PrP^{sc} selects the host PrP^{c} species closest to itself.

In the autocatalytic chain reaction, set up when PrP^{sc} converts PrP^{c} to PrP^{sc}, the products of both gene copies participate, and the more similar they are the more efficient is the reaction. This might explain why sporadic and iatrogenic CJD occur mainly in people in whom both copies of the PrP gene encode either methionine or valine at codon 129 (that is, homozygotes). People who carry one of each type of PrP gene (that is, heterozygotes) may be partially protected from prion disease because they produce two slightly different types of prion protein molecules which may interact less efficiently. The dynamics of this process may be such that in heterozygotes the chemical interaction rarely 'takes off', so the disease seldom occurs. In some families with inherited prion disease, the age at onset may be earlier in those family members who are homozygous at codon 129 because the disease progresses more efficiently when the products of both PrP gene copies participate fully in the disease process.

If the prion hypothesis is true, it follows that it should not be possible to transmit prion disease to an animal which does not have its own PrP^{c}. In 1992, Charles Weissmann and his colleagues in the Institute of Molecular Biology, Zurich, Switzerland reported that they had bred a mouse in which the PrP gene had been inactivated ('knocked out') and which lacked any PrP^{c}. It has not been possible to transmit mouse-adapted scrapie to such mice (Büeler *et al.* 1993). Similarly, Jean Manson and her colleagues in Edinburgh, using a slightly different technique, have produced mice which carry either two, one, or no copies of the mouse PrP gene (Manson *et al.* 1994). These mice have either the normal level of PrP^{c}, half the level of PrP^{c}, or no PrP^{c} in their brains. When injected intracerebrally with PrP^{sc} from mouse-adapted scrapie brain, those animals without PrP^{c} do not get sick, and those with half the normal PrP^{c} get sick after a much longer incubation period than those with the normal level of PrP^{c}.

The question has been raised as to whether in those families in which prion disease is associated with a mutation in the PrP gene, individuals become sick because they are susceptible to infection from an outside agent or because the disease is produced *de novo*. Again, scientists in Prusiner's laboratory have addressed this problem. Transgenic mice have been 'constructed' which carry multiple copies of a PrP gene with a mutation at codon 101, equivalent to the codon 102 proline-to-leucine mutation associated with human prion disease. These mice become ill *spontaneously* at about 160 days of age (Hsiao *et al.* 1990). Furthermore their brains show marked spongiform encephalopathy, and disease can be transmitted experimentally from these animals to other animals (Hsiao *et al.* 1994). In other words, a disease produced by a gene mutation gives rise to a transmissible agent. However, the interpretation of this experiment is not as clear-cut as at first it seems. The transgenic mice carried *multiple* copies of the mutant gene. In a similar experiment, Jean Manson and her colleagues in Edinburgh produced transgenic mice in which the normal mouse PrP gene was *replaced* by a copy containing the codon 101 proline-to-leucine mutation (Moore *et al.* 1995). These animals did not, therefore, carry multiple copies of the mutant gene. So far these animals have not developed disease spontaneously. Furthermore, Westaway and colleagues have produced a mouse which carries multiple copies of the *normal*, wild-type mouse PrP gene (Westaway *et al.* 1994*b*). These animals synthesize large amounts of PrP^c, and spontaneously develop a disease which includes muscle damage as well as brain damage. Spongiform encephalopathy is also experimentally transmissible from the brains of these mice (Prusiner 1994). More recently, Telling *et al.* (1996*a*) compared transgenic mice expressing only moderate but equal levels of either wild-type mouse PrP or 101 mutant PrP. Only the latter became sick, showing that the mutation, in addition to the level of PrP expression, is important in determining disease. The reader will discern from these experiments that there is still a long way to go before scientists can claim to understand fully the role of prion protein in the pathogenesis of prion diseases. In particular, experiments involving three sources of PrP—for example, donor tissue from one species injected into another species carrying transgenes from a third species—have produced very complex results. Most transgenic experiments now involve inserting PrP genes into mice whose own PrP gene has been deleted (PrP-null), which considerably simplifies the interpretation of results. Mice carrying chimeric transgenes, that is, inserted prion protein genes which consist of sequences from two species spliced together, have been used to explore the protein–protein interactions in the conversion of PrP^c to PrP^{sc}, and it is beginning to look as if other proteins might be involved in the conversion mechanism.

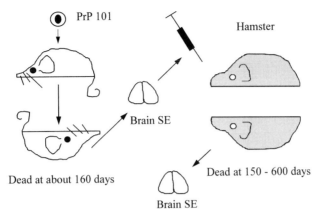

Fig 7.3 Experimental demonstration that a genetic disease can be transmitted to another animal. Transgenic mice carrying multiple copies of a mouse PrP gene in which position 101 is occupied by a leucine rather than the normal proline (equivalent to Pro102Leu in human GSS) became ill spontaneously at about 160 days of age. The brains showed spongiform change. Using the brains as donor tissue, disease could be transmitted to hamsters. The hamster brains also showed spongiform change. (After Hsiao *et al.* 1990, 1994.)

Transplants

In addition to creating transgenic mice, it is also possible to take live brain tissue from one mouse and transplant it into the brain of another mouse, where it will survive. The transplant will be genetically different from the host mouse. This system has been particularly useful where PrP transgenic brain tissue has been transplanted into the brains of PrP-null mice, so that the transplant contains lots of PrP^c while the rest of the brain contains none. Using this technique Charles Weissmann's group at the Institute of Molecular Biology teamed up with Adriano Aguzzi's group at the Institute of Neuropatholgy, both in Zurich, to demonstrate two remarkable features of prion disease. First, if a PrP-null mouse carrying a brain tissue transplant expressing PrP is injected in the brain with infectious tissue, spongiform encephalopathy will develop in the transplant (which will die), but the PrP-null host mouse will remain healthy. Large amounts of PrP^{sc} spill out from the transplant but do not cause spongiform encephalopathy or neuronal loss in the host mouse brain. This suggests that it is the process of conversion of PrP^c to PrP^{sc}, rather than the presence of PrP^{sc} itself, which is toxic to brain tissue (Brandner *et al.* 1996*a*). Secondly, if a PrP-null mouse carrying a PrP-expressing transplant is injected peripherally with infectious tissue, neither the host mouse nor the transplant will develop spongiform encephalopathy.

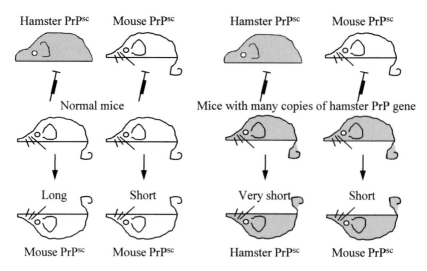

Fig. 7.4 A series of experiments in which transgenic mice have been used to illustrate the relationships between the infecting (donor) PrP^{sc} and the host PrP^{c}. When PrP^{sc} from hamster-adapted scrapie is injected intracerebrally into normal mice, the mice become sick after a long incubation time and the PrP^{sc} produced by the host is mouse PrP^{sc}. When mouse-adapted scrapie is injected into normal mice, the incubation time is short and, again, the PrP^{sc} produced in the host is mouse PrP^{sc}. The difference in incubation times is a measure of the species barrier. However, when hamster-adapted scrapie is injected into transgenic mice carrying a number of copies of the hamster PrP gene (such that the mice produce both hamster and mouse PrP^{c}), the species barrier is essentially abolished. The mice get sick after a very short incubation time and the PrP^{sc} produced in the host is hamster PrP^{sc}. When the same transgenic mice are injected with mouse-adapted scrapie, they also become sick and the PrP^{sc} produced in the host is mouse PrP^{sc}. In other words, hamster PrP^{sc} interacts exclusively with hamster PrP^{c} and mouse PrP^{sc} interacts exclusively with mouse PrP^{c} in these transgenic mice.

This suggests that PrP^{sc} does not travel around the body until it reaches the transplant. Rather infectivity seems to travel by converting PrP^{c} to PrP^{sc} along its route, somewhat like a chain of dominoes knocking each other down (Brandner *et al.* 1996*b*). The scientific community has high regard for elegant experiments like these.

Tissue cultures

Most experiments mentioned in the course of our discussion about prion diseases have involved animals. Experimental transmissions of spongiform encephalopathy consist, usually, of injecting brain homogenate from an affected animal (or human) directly into the brain of another suitable animal and waiting for disease to develop.

In addition to the use of live animals, cell cultures have also been used in the study of the conversion mechanism. Cell cultures (or tissue cultures as they are also known) are prepared by collecting cells of interest from an animal (or human) and 'growing' them in a nutrient medium in a suitable container. Growing means allowing the cells in the culture to continue to divide. It may be necessary to transform these cells (in effect render them cancerous) in order to get them to grow continuously. Once a cell line is established in tissue culture it is possible to alter the genetic make-up of the cells by inserting genes (technically, transfecting them with altered genes). This is analogous to developing transgenic animals. Byron Caughey and his colleagues at the Rocky Mountain Laboratory in Montana, together with a number of other scientists, have been able to infect cultures of mouse neuroblastoma cells (cancerous nerve cells) which make PrP^c, with hamster-adapted scrapie, and to maintain the infectivity indefinitely. In other words, the cultured cells can facilitate the conversion of their own PrP^c to PrP^{sc}. These cell cultures are being used widely to examine which parts of the PrP^c molecule are necessary for conversion to the abnormal, protease K resistant form. Transgenic cell cultures carrying mutant PrP genes have been found to produce PrP which has many of the properties of PrP^{sc}, although it has yet to be shown to be infectious (Lehmann and Harris 1996).

Perhaps the most exciting experiments have been carried out in cell-free systems, that is, in real test tubes containing only those ingredients specified by the experimenter. If PrP^{sc} can act as a template or catalyst in the conversion of PrP^c molecules to PrP^{sc} molecules, and if all the information necessary for this reaction is contained within the structure of these molecules, can this be demonstrated in a cell-free system which does not contain all the biosynthetic mechanisms of normal cells? The answer appears to be yes. Byron Caughey, David Kocisko, and their colleagues at the Rocky Mountain Laboratory, in collaboration with Peter Lansbury from the Massachusetts Institute of Technology in Boston, have developed a cell-free system that converts PrP^c to PrP^{sc} (Caughey et al. 1996). They set up a cell culture which produces normal PrP^c. Furthermore, they grew these cells in a nutrient medium that included a radioactively labelled amino acid. Consequently, the PrP^c produced by this cell culture was radioactively labelled. This meant it could be detected by a radioactivity counting or measuring device. They extracted the radioactive PrP^c from the cell culture and mixed it with non-radioactive PrP^{sc} extracted from a scrapie-infected animal brain. After treating this mixture with various chemicals, they were able to show that the mixture now contained some radioactive PrP^{sc}. In other words it seems that some of the PrP^c had been converted to PrP^{sc}. Since all this had been done without living cells being involved, it implied that the increase in the amount of PrP^{sc} was the result of a chemical reaction rather than the influence of a micro-organism. If this experiment was carried out without the PrP^{sc} from the infected animal brain being added to the mixture, there was no conversion of radioactive PrP^c to radioactive PrP^{sc}. This was direct evidence that the abnormal form of the prion protein was acting as a catalyst or template for the conversion of normal prion protein to the abnormal form.

Unfortunately these researchers were unable to determine whether or not the radioactive PrP^{sc} was infectious because in this reaction the amount of added non-radioactive PrP^{sc} was far in excess of the radioactive PrP^{sc} produced, so any additional infectivity was swamped. Nevertheless, this important experiment, published in *Nature*, opened the way to exploring the basis of the old problem for the prion hypothesis, strains of agent.

The challenge of strain of agent

Scientists who reject the prion hypothesis argue that the infectious agent in prion disease must contain a nucleic acid genome. They regard the agent as an independent, replicating organism which infects the host in a more or less conventional way. They argue that PrP is merely a factor, in the host, through which the agent operates, such that the symptoms seen in the host will be influenced by variations in the PrP gene that the host carries. Apart from transmissibility itself, the most cogent evidence put forward for the existence of an independent, infectious agent has been the phenomenon known as 'strain of agent'. Conventional viruses, such as that which causes influenza, exist in slightly different genetic forms or strains, each causing disease with slightly different symptoms. In prion disease the strain of agent is defined by the length of the incubation period (time from infection to sickness) and the lesion profile (distribution of pathology across different parts of the brain) in the affected animal. This, of course, is a feature of the infected animal, but since the agent is 'invisible', it is the nearest it is possible to get to the agent itself. The response of the animal to the agent depends, not surprisingly, on the PrP gene in the animal. There are two forms of the PrP gene in mice. Most mice carry two copies of one type of PrP gene called PrP-a, while other mice carry two copies of PrP-b. (Cross-bred mice carry one copy of each.) Roughly speaking, isolates of scrapie, taken from sheep with naturally occurring scrapie, when injected into mice will produce disease which has either a short incubation period in PrP-a/PrP-a mice and a long incubation in PrP-b/PrP-b mice, or vice versa, depending on source of scrapie isolate. As disease (and thus agent) is transmitted back and forth between mice of the two types, strains of agent emerge which have an affinity for one type of mouse or the other. When transmitted out of, and into, their preferred type of mouse, the agent produces a stable and short incubation time, but when it is passed to the other type of mouse it becomes unstable and may change its properties to such an extent that it is, in effect, a new strain.

These data indicate that, in order to predict how long the incubation period will be, one needs to know not only the type of mouse *to which* disease is being transmitted (known as the host) but also the type of mouse *from which* the disease is being transmitted (known as the donor). It turns out that even this is not enough. Sometimes agent from different original sources (for example two scrapie-affected sheep) will produce different incubation periods in one type of mouse (for example, PrP-a/PrP-a mice), even when they have both been transmitted through intermediate mice of the same type (also, for example, PrP-a/PrP-a mice). This difference in incubation period is attributed to something in the agent which is independent of the prion protein in either the host or the donor. It has been argued that only nucleic acid can carry the sort of information that could produce this sort of variation and that, therefore, the agent must be an independent organism with its own genes, made of nucleic acid. In our view this is not an obligatory interpretation of the data. Moira Bruce and Hugh Fraser of the Neuropathogenesis Unit in Edinburgh, where work on scrapie has been carried out for many years, claim that there are at least 20 strains of mouse-adapted scrapie (Fraser *et al.* 1989), but we believe that variation in the PrP gene of the host and donor mice has *not* been fully taken into account in arriving at this calculation, and that the number of separate strains may be considerably less than 20, and quite possibly as few as two or three (Ridley and Baker 1996b). None the less, there is undoubtedly a source of variation which is not determined by the primary amino acid sequence of the PrP protein of the host or donor. It is our view that this information could be carried in the *shape* or *conformation* that the PrP^{sc} molecules adopt, but as yet this possibility remains unproved, and we might be wrong (Ridley and Baker 1997).

One of the ways in which it can be decided whether strains of agent exist because of variation in nucleic acid in the agent is to see whether strains are preserved in the cell-free conversion experiments described above. If strain differences are preserved, they cannot be due to variation in nucleic acid in the agent because nucleic acid cannot replicate under the conditions of these experiments. Transmissible mink encephalopathy (TME) has been transmitted to hamsters and, following further transmission from hamster to hamster (of the same genetic background), two characteristic patterns of disease presentation emerge. This has been interpreted as evidence for two strains of TME agent. One strain, 'drowsy', causes the hamsters to become sleepy, while the other, 'hyper', causes the hamsters to become overactive. Eventually, of course, all the animals succumb to a spongiform encephalopathy. Caughey and his colleagues used these strains of hamster-adapted TME in cell-free conversion experiments and the radioactive PrP^{sc} produced was found to have the same characteristics as the strain of agent that had been used to trigger the conversion (Bessen et al. 1995).

The issue of strain of agent is very important, not only because it challenges the prion hypothesis with data that the hypothesis has difficulty explaining, but also because certain trends in the behaviour of agent strains have implications for identifying the origin of different types of prion disease. Prion disease is an endemic disease (continuously occurring at a low level) only in sheep and humans. Different isolates of sheep scrapie (that is, scrapie isolated from brains of different sheep) frequently generate disease in mice indicative of different strains, and the unpredictableness with which human prion disease will transmit to mice suggests that human disease also produces many different strains of agent. BSE is the only epidemic prion disease (where lots of cases are related to the same events) to have been studied in detail. Isolates of BSE from several different cows, and from cats and zoo animals which developed a spongiform encephalopathy during the BSE epidemic and which had presumably been infected by the same contaminated material, all seemed to contain the same single strain of BSE agent (Bruce et al. 1994). One year after the report of the new variant of CJD in Britain, the results of 'strain typing' of material from these patients were anxiously awaited, since this would cast light on the supposition that their disease was a consequence of eating contaminated meat products.

Preservation of strain in human prion disease

In humans a mutation at codon 178 of the PrP gene (aspartic acid to asparagine) is associated with prion disease. As we discussed in an earlier chapter, the form of the disease depends on what is encoded at codon 129 (the common polymorphic site) on the mutant copy, irrespective of what codon 129 encodes on the other copy. If the patient carries PrP178 asparagine with 129 methionine, the prion disease will present as fatal familial insomnia (FFI). The disease is characterized by marked insomnia, which is resistant to treatment, together with a general breakdown in a number of physiological functions, leading eventually to death. Post-mortem examination of the brain shows that the thalamus (a large nucleus within the brain) is affected. It is atrophied (shrunken) and there is some spongiform encephalopathy. PrP^{sc} can be extracted from the brain, although it is there in small amounts. If, on the other hand, the patient carries PrP178 asparagine with 129 valine, the clinical presentation is CJD-like. In these individuals the brain shows marked spongiform encephalopathy, and PrP^{sc} can be extracted. It turns out that after digestion of the FFI-PrP^{sc} with proteinase K, the remaining protein fragment has a molecular weight of 19 kilodaltons; after treating the CJD-PrP^{sc} in the same way the remaining protein fragment has a molecular weight of 21 kilodaltons. FFI and CJD resulting from the mutation at codon 178 of the PrP gene can be thought of as giving rise to different strains of PrP^{sc}, and that the difference is determined by the common polymorphism at codon 129. This raises the question of whether the strain difference would be preserved on transmission to a suitable host. Unfortunately this type of CJD or FFI is difficult to transmit to mice. However, it is possible to create new genes which are chimeric, that is, made of a mixture of parts of the mouse PrP gene and parts of the PrP gene from another species (Prusiner et al. 1990). These genes can then be inserted into a mouse to make a transgenic, chimeric mouse. Glenn Telling and colleagues in Prusiner's laboratory have investigated the question of strain preservation in FFI/CJD in a series of elegant experiments using transgenic mice carrying copies of a chimeric mouse–human PrP gene (consisting of a sequence of the human PrP gene sandwiched between two mouse PrP gene sequences) (Telling et al. 1996b). These mice produce chimeric mouse–human PrP^c. When disease was transmitted to these transgenic mice using extracts of brain from FFI patients, the proteinase K resistant fragment of the chimeric mouse–human PrP^{sc} produced had a molecular weight of 19 kilodaltons; when brain extracts from CJD patients were used to infect the mice, the resistant fragment had a molecular weight of 21 kilodaltons. These authors concluded that their results 'suggest a mechanism to explain strains of prions where diversity is encrypted in the conformation of PrP^{sc}'.

Which bits of the PrP molecule are interacting?

The mouse and hamster PrP genes differ at about 16 codons. If a transgenic mouse is constructed so that its PrP gene has two hamster codons, the gene continues to behave like a mouse PrP gene, but if it has five hamster codons, it behaves like a hamster PrP gene. Transgenic mice carrying the two-substitution genes are resistant to hamster-adapted agent, whereas mice carrying the five-substitution genes are susceptible to both hamster-adapted and mouse-adapted agent (Prusiner 1997). Even more interesting is the observation that the infectious agent generated from these five-substitution chimeric mice is capable of infecting *both* mice and hamsters. The agent is therefore behaving differently from mouse-adapted and hamster-adapted strains of agent, and could be regarded as a new strain of agent. By making many different chimeric genes, which differ at different codons, it is possible, after many painstaking experiments, using thousands of mice, to work out exactly how the PrP molecules interact to produce the species-barrier effects (that is, the difficulty in transmitting disease from one species to another) that are observed experimentally. All this might seem terribly academic were it not for the fact that the species barrier is the only thing that really protects us from BSE.

8

Down on the farm: BSE

As we reached the end of 1996, it was announced that Britain was to go ahead with a 'selective cull' of something like 100 000 healthy cattle. It is most unlikely that these animals were destined to become sick but, in order to reassure its fellow Europeans that they would definitely not become sick, the Government decided to kill them. Between April and December of that year about a million healthy cattle over 30 months of age, which had outlived their economic usefulness as dairy cows or breeding animals, had already been slaughtered and their carcasses destroyed to prevent them from being eaten. There can be few people in Britain who have not seen news film of dead cows being shovelled into massive incinerators. All this death and destruction was the aftermath of the worst calamity ever to have befallen the British food and farming industry. Bovine spongiform encephalopathy, BSE, or, to give it the name by which it is better known and which has added the spice to so many hysterical newspaper headlines, 'mad cow disease', has cost the Britain Government about £3 billion or $5 billion in compensation, disposal costs, and other expenses over the past decade. The cost to farming and the many associated industries is incalculable. At the end of 1996, the ban on the export of all bovine products from Britain to anywhere in the world, imposed by the European Commission, was still in place, and there was little evidence that it would be lifted in the near future. The selective cull would be nothing more than a ritual sacrifice, a political gesture, by which the UK Government would attempt to placate its European partners in the hope that the ban would be eased. All those who had spent the past decade trying to understand this dreadful disease knew that there was no scientific reason for killing these animals, a view shared by the then Agriculture Minister, Douglas Hogg. Interviewed on the 'Today' programme on BBC Radio 4 on Tuesday, 17 December 1996, Hogg said that at a meeting of European Heads of State, held in Florence some months before, it was agreed that Britain would carry out a selective cull of those unaffected cattle that, it was thought, might be at some risk of contracting BSE, in order to speed up the end of the epidemic. Further scientific analysis of the epidemic suggested that this cull would make little, if any, impact on the course of the epidemic, and plans for the cull were suspended. This angered the other European Member States who insisted that there would be no lifting of the ban if the selective cull was not carried out. Hogg told the radio interviewer that he and colleagues still believed that there were no scientific grounds for carrying out the slaughter, but that Britain had to do so if there was going to be any chance of getting the ban lifted. So what brought the country to this dreadful position?

Beginnings

It is difficult to be certain exactly when the first cow to get BSE became sick. It is possible that a very few animals had died with BSE before the disease came to the attention of the veterinary services. We do know that in April 1985 a veterinary surgeon was called to a farm in the south of England to see an adult Friesian-Holstein (black-and-white) cow. This normally placid animal had become hypersensitive to noise, apprehensive, unpredictable, and aggressive, and was having difficulty walking. Two common disorders of dairy cows in the UK could have produced these symptoms— hypomagnesaemia and nervous ketosis—but this cow did not respond to treatments for these conditions. Eventually it was put down and its brain was sent to the Central Veterinary Laboratory (CVL) at Weybridge in Surrey for examination by veterinary neuropathologist Gerald Wells. Over the following 12 months, several more dairy cows developed similar clinical signs and, for each, the course of illness progressed over 1–5 months. The brains of these animals, together with those from a number of similarly afflicted animals from other herds, were also examined by Gerald Wells and his colleagues, who were beginning to see a pattern of pathology reminiscent of that seen in scrapie-affected sheep. Chemical extraction of the brains yielded fibrils similar to those that could be extracted from scrapie-affected sheep (scrapie-associated fibrils, or SAFs) and which were considered diagnostic of scrapie. A full and consistent clinical picture was assembled which, with the equally consistent neuropathological changes, led to a growing confidence that this was a new disease. The report of their findings began with a somewhat understated lead paragraph: 'In routine diagnostic submissions to their laboratories the authors have recently recognised an encephalopathy associated with a novel clinical syndrome in cattle from dairy herds in widely separated geographical locations of England' (Wells *et al.* 1987).

When a definitive diagnosis had been made on only six cows, alarm bells sounded, and veterinary scientists decided that they had to know the extent of this disease. An epidemiological investigation into BSE was started in June 1987. Little did anyone know that even by that time at least 50 000 cows destined to develop BSE had already become infected, and that over the following 10 years more than 160 000 animals were to succumb to the disease. CVL epidemiologists later calculated that, for each animal showing signs of BSE, at least two further animals had been infected but did not live long enough to get the disease, probably because they were slaughtered for food. This may have been an underestimate. In a detailed analysis of the epidemic, published in mid-1996, a group of Oxford researchers argued that, although 160 000 animals had died from BSE during the previous 10 years, a further 700 000 animals had been infected. So, even before Gerald Wells's report of the new disease was published, it is likely that there may have been as many as 200 000 infected cattle in the UK. But no one could have known this, since only a handful of these cows had developed symptoms and died.

What was the cause?

The Ministry of Agriculture, Fisheries and Food (MAFF), through its Veterinary Investigation (VI) Centres and the Central Veterinary Laboratory, set about the detective work necessary to answer this question. Under the leadership of John Wilesmith, the small veterinary epidemiology department at CVL began the laborious task of collecting information on all suspected cases of BSE referred to VI centres throughout the country. At this stage (June 1987) such referrals were voluntary. The data were collected by means of a detailed questionnaire which covered date of birth of the affected animal, sex, breed, herd of origin, date of onset of illness, and much more, including the age structure of the herds, whether there had been sheep on the farm, details of vaccines, etc. There were questions relating to the clinical signs seen in the animals and the progression of the illness. There were also questions about the feeding practices. Although this questionnaire has been modified, and BSE was made a notifiable disease in June 1988, this method of data collection has been used throughout the

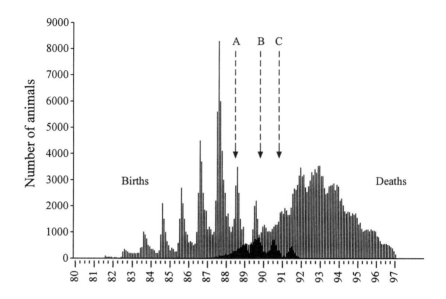

Fig. 8.1 The BSE epidemic up to March 1997. The number of animals dying with BSE reached a peak in 1993 and declined rapidly thereafter. The left-hand part of the graph illustrates the birth distribution of those animals that went on to develop BSE. This distribution shows annual fluctuations because of the time of year at which calves are born, and the fact that calves born in the winter months are fed more supplementary feedstuffs than those born during the summer, when grass is more plentiful. The 5-year difference between the peaks of the two distributions is a measure of the average incubation time from infection shortly after birth to death at age 4–5 years. There was a marked drop in the number of animals destined to get BSE which were born after the introduction of the Ruminant Feed Ban (A), and a further reduction after the Specified Offals Ban was put in place (B). The Specified Offals Ban was subsequently extended to cover all animals, including pigs and poultry (C). Few cows born after 1992 will get BSE.

epidemic, and CVL now has a very extensive and complex database. Initially, the aim of the survey was to obtain data from 200 cases of BSE, and this was achieved by the end of 1987 (Wilesmith *et al.* 1988). The Central Veterinary Laboratory has produced many papers over the years, describing all aspects of the BSE epidemic. These have been published in a variety of journals but readers should be aware that there is often a long time between submission of a report for publication and its appearance in print, which in some cases can be as long as a year, so that the published information may give an indication of the state of knowledge many months earlier.

Early epidemiological findings

In their early reports, John Wilesmith and his colleagues confirmed and extended the descriptions of the clinical signs of BSE. The most common feature described by farmers was a change in behaviour. Animals were 'nervous' about going into the milking parlours, were hyper-responsive to touch, and tended to kick when being handled. Initially, there were subtle abnormalities in walking ability, leading eventually to obvious difficulties in maintaining balance. This was most apparent when an animal had to move about on the slippery concrete floor of a pen, and a film of Daisy, an early sufferer from BSE, in such a predicament has often been shown on television. Other signs included loss of weight and reduction in milk yields. For most cases the duration of the illness was between 1 and 2 months, although it could vary from less than 1 month to as long as 7 or 8 months, and there were animals whose illness lasted for a year or so. However, it was difficult to estimate the duration of illness with any accuracy since most animals were put down because of their repeated falling.

In trying to establish the cause of BSE from their epidemiological investigations, Wilesmith's team were able to rule out a number of possibilities. They reported that there were no specific, common factors in the treatment of calves, young animals, or adult animals (including vaccinations, organophosphorous fly treatments, hormones, or treatments for parasitic worms), which applied only to affected animals and which might have led to those animals developing BSE. They also argued that the disease was not a simple genetic disease and that, since the neuropathological picture resembled that of scrapie, BSE was probably caused by exposure to a transmissible agent similar to, or identical to, the one associated with scrapie in sheep. Furthermore, the age distribution of affected animals suggested that exposure to this agent probably started about 1981/82. As they were preparing their report, Wilesmith and colleagues learned that Hugh Fraser at the Neuropathogenesis Unit in Edinburgh had successfully induced a spongiform encephalopathy in mice following intracerebral injection of brain homogenate from a BSE-affected cow, and this added weight to the argument. The way in which new cases were appearing suggested an 'extended common source epidemic', that is, an epidemic in which every affected animal acquires the agent in the same way from the same source (for as long as the source is available) and in which there is no direct animal-to-animal transmission of disease. The possibility that BSE resulted from contact with scrapie-affected sheep, either by direct animal-to-animal contact or by shared pasture, was ruled out. Wilesmith concluded that the most likely route of contamination was via cattle feedstuffs, pointing out that there was a precedent for this in the outbreaks of transmissible mink encephalopathy, which had occurred in mink farms in the United States. In these small epidemics it was accepted that mink had become ill as a result of eating some meat or animal-derived feedstuff, of which scrapie-affected sheep was one possibility, although this has never been proved.

Cattle are fed commercially prepared feed supplements during the winter months when there is little grass. Dairy cows, needing lots of protein to sustain the production of lots of milk, are fed more supplements than beef cattle. Dairy herds had a much higher incidence of BSE than did beef herds. It was beginning to look as though the supplementary feedstuffs could be the source of infection. These feedstuffs contain protein concentrates which are prepared from the rendered carcasses of dead animals.

Where does cattle feed come from?

Before the BSE epidemic entered our lives, rendering and related activities did not impinge on public awareness, but it has been impossible to escape news reports illustrating just how unsavoury, though necessary, the industry is. Animal carcasses are collected and 'cooked' at high temperatures in large ovens to yield two products, meat-and-bone meal and tallow (fat). During the processing, organic solvents are used to increase the amount of fat recovered and the solvents are subsequently removed by heat treatment. Although tallow is also used in feed supplements, epidemiological data suggested that it was not a significant source of infection and that the meat-and-bone meal was much more likely to be the source of the problem. The underlying hypothesis, of course, was that the scrapie agent in affected sheep carcasses had survived the rendering process and had contaminated the meat-and-bone meal, a powdery, protein-rich product subsequently incorporated into feed supplements. At about this time reports were also appearing about a spongiform encephalopathy in zoo animals, the first concerning a nyala and a gemsbok. These animals were in different collections and had had no contact with each other. Their illness was discovered during routine screening and at first a genetic explanation was considered. This idea was soon abandoned. These animals had been fed on commercially produced feedstuffs which did not normally contain animal-derived meat-and-bone meal, making use of soya protein instead. However, a rapid increase in the price of soya had brought about the inclusion of animal meat-and-bone meal in the diet of these animals for a short period of time, and it seems that this short exposure was sufficient to bring about the disease in these animals.

Why Guernsey but not Jersey?

In the early days of the epidemic, BSE appeared on the Channel Island of Guernsey but not on the island of Jersey. Both have substantial dairy herds and, although the manufacturers of the cattle feedstuffs used in these two islands were different, they were both in mainland Great Britain. Feedstuffs were not imported from any other source. Eventually, BSE did appear in Jersey, but at a much lower level than in Guernsey. The paradox was resolved, providing further evidence for a feedborne source of infection, when investigations revealed that the feedstuff supplier to Guernsey used a lot of meat-and-bone meal whereas the supplier to Jersey used far less.

Why then?

Meat-and-bone meal has been used in cattle rations for many years, not only in the UK but throughout Europe and the USA. Yet it seemed that meat-and-bone meal was becoming contaminated in the UK, possibly as a result of a change in the way in which it was manufactured. John Wilesmith listed a number of factors that may have been important. For example, there was a gradual increase in the sheep population of Great Britain during the 1970s and 1980s and there was probably an increase in the number of sheep with scrapie going into the rendering process. Until 1994, scrapie was not a notifiable disease and the true prevalence of the disease (the number of animals affected at any time) was not known with accuracy. Farmers were reluctant to admit to scrapie. It is certainly true that the UK has had a problem with scrapie for years, with levels higher than in the rest of Europe or the USA. Wilesmith also pointed out that, as a result of a decline in the number of knacker's yards, more sheep condemned as unfit for human consumption and sheep dying in accidents were being included in the rendering process, and that more sheep heads were being rendered. These are all important factors which may go some way to explaining why meat-and-bone meal should have become contaminated. More importantly, there had been changes in the rendering processes. In the late 1970s, the rendering industry moved from the less efficient batchwise method of dealing with material to a continuous process, a sort of conveyor-belt system. As the price of fat fell throughout the world, the use of organic solvents in fat extraction was reduced, and, since operating at the high temperatures necessary for the removal of solvents is expensive, the processing temperatures could then be lowered and duration of heat treatment could be shortened. Most researchers accept that these changes in the rendering process allowed more of the scrapie agent from sheep to escape inactivation and some agent to be passed to cattle via meat-and-bone meal. However, there are a few problems with this view.

First, is not clear that the scrapie agent was inactivated by the 'old' rendering processes before the changes were made at the beginning of the 1980s. In the old batch rendering methods, material to be rendered was chopped into small pieces, about 4 inches (10 cm) cubed, and then cooked for 90–120 minutes, achieving a temperature somewhere between 100 and 150°C, after which the fat was skimmed from the top. Professor Richard Lacey has reported that some infectivity can survive 360°C for 60 minutes. He describes a number of newer continuous methods and the temperatures achieved by those methods, and does not believe that either the old batch processing or the newer continuous processing is certain to inactivate the scrapie or BSE agents (Lacey 1994). Lacey, Professor of Clinical Microbiology at the University of Leeds, has been a controversial figure in matters of public health, especially in relation to food hygiene. He drew to public attention the risks of listeriosis (a bacterial disease associated with the contamination of dairy products such as cheese) in pregnancy and, when BSE appeared, joined with his colleague Dr Stephen Dealler, in proposing that all cattle in the UK should be slaughtered, to prevent the disease reaching epidemic proportions. He has appeared on radio and television programmes many times, arguing that the Government has been operating a cover-up of the facts about BSE, and on a number of occasions has suggested that many hundreds of thousands of people may die as a result of eating BSE-affected meat. His book *Mad cow disease: the history of BSE in Britain* (Lacey 1994) is his view of the BSE story, a view not shared by everyone. Secondly, other countries have changed their rendering processes in a similar way and BSE has not been reported in these countries, although these countries may have much lower levels of scrapie. Thirdly, the underlying assumption of the feedstuff hypothesis is that scrapie agent, having survived rendering, will cause disease if eaten by cattle. However, surprising as it may seem, experiments to demonstrate that disease can be experimentally transmitted to cattle following feeding of feedstuff contaminated with known amounts of infected sheep brain have not, to our knowledge, been attempted. Finally, the BSE agent is different from all known strains of scrapie agent. Since the group of scientists at the Neuropathogenesis Unit in Edinburgh, who specialize in describing strain differences, have argued that the BSE strain does not change when it is transmitted from one animal to another and has not been found in sheep, we are left with something of a mystery as to the origin of this agent. Of course, after the beginning of the epidemic, cattle with BSE would also have gone into the rendering process and contributed to the contamination of the meat-and-bone meal. The accidental transmission of prion disease is at its most efficient when the donor and recipient animals are of the same species, so when affected cattle entered the rendering process the epidemic must have been established. Few people doubt that the year-on-year increase in the birth of cattle that went on to get BSE from 1985 to 1988 was due to recycling of the BSE agent, but whether BSE came originally from scrapie, from a very low level of BSE occurring in cattle before 1986, or from elsewhere may never be known. It is quite possible that the BSE epidemic had its origin in a single spontaneous case in a cow which then entered the rendering process. If the rate of spontaneously arising disease in cattle was the same as in humans, at about one per million of the population per year, it might go unnoticed, since most animals would be slaughtered before clinical signs appeared. If just one animal with a prion disease survived long enough to develop high levels of infectivity and then was rendered by a process which was inefficient at destroying the agent, the infectivity could spread via the meat-and-bone to other animals. There is a clear analogy here with some views on the origin of kuru. But it is much easier to work out how a disease is maintained than it is to work out where it came from in the first place, as those researching the AIDS epidemic have discovered.

Proving the hypothesis

During the first few months of 1988, CVL investigators contacted feedstuff manufacturers about the inclusion rates of meat-and-bone meal in their products and used this information to check the feeding history of affected cattle. This exercise substantiated the hypothesis that the epidemic was being caused by contaminated feedstuff. Further epidemiological analysis using case-control methods, in which 'cases' (BSE-affected animals) are each paired with 'controls' (unaffected animals of the same age) in order to investigate differences between each animal in a pair, indicated that a large proportion of all BSE cases was probably exposed to the infectious agent during the first 6 months of life. The reason for this is that the likelihood of a cow developing BSE depended to some extent on what time of year it was born. Calves are fed more supplementary feedstuffs if they are born during the winter than if they are born in the summer, when they can be put out on grass at a younger age.

Early responses to the epidemic

In April 1988, the Minister of Agriculture, Fisheries and Food and the Secretary of State for Health jointly appointed a small working party of scientists to look at the BSE problem and to make recommendations to ministers about what should be done. The committee was chaired by Professor Sir Richard Southwood, an eminent Oxford zoologist, and included three other distinguished, but retired, scientists. The choice of committee members was surprising since none had ever worked in the field of spongiform encephalopathy. They relied for their information on John Wilesmith, who was attached to the committee as advisor. Even before the Southwood Committee held its first meeting, the Government put legislation in place to make BSE a notifiable disease and to ban the feeding to ruminants (cattle and sheep) of feedstuff containing any protein derived from ruminants (excluding milk, milk products, and calcium-rich supplements prepared from bone). BSE became notifiable on 21 June 1988, and the Ruminant Feed Ban came into force one month later on 21 July. Even though the evidence that BSE was caused by contaminated feedstuff was compelling, this delay of a month was intended to allow stocks of feedstuff containing ruminant-derived protein to be used up. This may sound extraordinary, but it must be appreciated that the supply of, and trade in, animals and perishable goods is extremely complicated. An alternative source of animal feedstuff had to be established. Rash legislation leads to wild swings in the availability of products, and people anxious to feed their animals might well resort to unconventional methods which could be hazardous to animal and ultimately human health. None the less, the Ruminant Feed Ban began when the number of animals becoming infected was climbing very rapidly, so it is likely that this month-long delay allowed several thousand more animals to become infected. Other measures were also put in place including, for example, the requirement that BSE-affected, pregnant animals had to be isolated when calving, and for 3 days afterwards, to minimize the risk of transmitting disease to other animals. This was based on the assumption (probably incorrect) that BSE might be transmitted via the placenta.

At its first meeting, the Southwood Committee immediately welcomed the imposition of the Ruminant Feed Ban and advised the Government that all BSE-affected animals should be identified and the carcasses destroyed. Although the Government received this advice in mid-June, such a requirement was not introduced until August, in order to work out a suitable procedure. The farmer was required to inform a veterinary surgeon that an animal might have BSE. The animal was killed and the brain removed for neuropathological examination and, if diagnosis was confirmed, the farmer was paid 50 per cent of the animal's value in compensation. If diagnosis was not confirmed, the farmer was paid the full value. The compensation for a confirmed case was later increased to 100 per cent because some people had argued that suspect cases were not being reported. When compensation was increased, there was no effect on the number of cases notified, suggesting that BSE had not been greatly under-reported. Up to the time the Southwood Committee made its recommendation that the carcasses of BSE-affected cattle be destroyed, meat from such animals had probably been used for human food. There was, and still is, no evidence that the consumption of meat from scrapie-affected sheep can lead to disease in humans, and the assumption was made by most scientists at that time that, if BSE was similar to scrapie, meat from BSE-affected cattle was unlikely to pose a risk to humans.

The Ruminant Feed Ban, which had initially been a temporary measure, was made permanent in November 1988, and by the end of that year, the use of milk from suspect cattle was prohibited for any purpose other than feeding to the cow's own calf. By the end of 1988 some 2000 animals had been confirmed as having BSE.

The first full report of the Southwood Committee was published in February 1989. It made a number of further recommendations, all of which were eventually implemented. These included the setting up of a scientific committee under the chairmanship of a virologist, Dr David Tyrrell. Other members included: Professor John Bourne, Director of the Institute for Animal Health; Dr Richard Kimberlin, a private consultant on scrapie-like diseases who had worked at the Neuropathogenesis Unit (NPU) in Edinburgh; Dr Bill Watson, Director of the Central Veterinary Laboratory; and Dr Bob Will, Consultant Neurologist in Edinburgh. Watson and Kimberlin had worked on scrapie for many years and Kimberlin, in particular, had been at the centre of opposition to the prion hypothesis. Bob Will, a charming Scotsman, had earlier carried out an epidemiological study of CJD in England and Wales. It should come as no surprise, therefore, that, when the Tyrrell Committee recommended that a unit be set up to monitor the number of cases of CJD in Britain and to determine whether there were any changes in the incidence, Will was chosen to head the unit. The Tyrrell Committee later became the Spongiform Encephalopathy Advisory Committee (SEAC). It is of interest to note that until John Collinge joined SEAC some years later no one on either the Tyrrell or SEAC committees subscribed to the prion hypothesis.

Other measures that stemmed from the Southwood Committee included the Specified Bovine Offals (SBO) Ban (part 1) which came into force in November 1989, and which prohibited the use in human food of brain, spinal cord, and certain other offals from all bovine animals over the age of 6 months, whether affected with BSE or not. This was the major component of government action to protect human health. In BSE-affected cattle, infectivity is found almost exclusively in brain and spinal cord, with possible infectivity in the other specified offals. By banning these tissues in human food, irrespective of whether the cow appeared to be ill, it was intended to exclude contamination from cows which were incubating the disease but which seemed to be well. Infectivity rises throughout the course of the incubation period and is only detectable in brain shortly before the onset of symptoms, but the SBO Ban prevented the consumption of these tissues from all cattle over 6 months of age. The SBO Ban was extended (part 2) almost a year later to prohibit the use of specified bovine offals in any animal food in order to prevent ruminant-derived protein (still in use in feedstuff for non-ruminant farm animals such as pigs and poultry) from being inadvertently fed to cattle. The SBO Ban was later extended to include tissues from calves under 6 months of age as well as some other tissues.

Was BSE experimentally transmissible?

At the beginning of the BSE epidemic scientists could only guess at the true nature of the disease and could not predict with any accuracy what the extent of the epidemic would be. These concerns, in 1986/1987, would be reflected in similar concerns about the new variant form of CJD some 10 years later. Southwood's first report, for example, taking into account the results of Wilesmith's early epidemiological data which suggested that exposure to contaminated feedstuff started in 1981/1982 and assumed that the level of exposure was constant between that time and the Ruminant Feed Ban, concluded:

if the age structure of the national adult herd remains constant, as the usual life span of a milk cow in Great Britain is at present 5 to 6 years this rate of presentation of the disease will continue until 1993, a cumulative total of about 17 000–20 000 cases from cows currently alive and subclinically infected. Thereafter, if cattle-to-cattle transmission does not occur then a reduction in incidence would follow with a very low incidence in 1996 and the subsequent disappearance of the disease.

The number of animals to die from BSE was underestimated by a factor of 10, although the estimate of the duration of the epidemic is turning out to be fairly accurate.

Although it appeared in 1986 that BSE belonged to the group of spongiform encephalopathies or prion diseases, experiments were set up to establish that it was experimentally transmissible. Most of these experiments involved mice, but one experiment was set up to compare the transmissibility of scrapie and BSE to primates. In the autumn of 1988, it was reported that BSE could be transmitted to mice following intracerebral injection of affected cattle brain homogenate, and early in 1990 cattle-to-cattle transmission following intracerebral injection and intravenous injection of BSE brain homogenate was reported. Perhaps more newsworthy was the demonstration that BSE could be transmitted to mice by the oral route, that is by feeding mice on a mash containing raw BSE-affected cattle brain. Some scientists suggest that oral administration of infectious agent is 100 000 times less efficient in transmitting disease than direct introduction of agent into the brain.

Could BSE be transmitted to primates? Would BSE transmit to primates any more readily than did scrapie? We were in a position to answer these questions. In conjunction with Gerald Wells at the Central Veterinary Laboratory, we set up experiments early in 1988, involving four marmosets (small New World monkeys) born and bred in our laboratory. Although a number of transmission experiments involving rodents had already been set up by others, they were still in progress and there was still no direct evidence that BSE was a transmissible disease. Brain tissue was collected from a recently killed BSE-affected cow and from a Greyface sheep which had suffered from scrapie. The tissue was homogenized and we injected two marmosets intracerebrally with the BSE tissue and the other two with the scrapie tissue. The injection was carried out under a general anaesthetic after which the monkeys recovered quickly and behaved perfectly normally.

None of the animals showed any sign of illness for almost 4 years. Then one of the scrapie-injected animals began to exhibit subtle neurological signs. It seemed to have difficulty keeping its balance and was unable to hold its slice of banana in both hands during feeding, preferring instead to leave it on the floor and to chew from it. Eventually, all animals became ill and were killed in line with the UK Home Office Project Licence under which the experiments were carried out. The brains were examined by Gerald Wells at CVL, and he confirmed that all four animals had a spongiform encephalopathy. The animals injected with scrapie tissue had survived for 41 months and those injected with BSE had survived 48 months. We concluded that brain tissue from BSE-affected cattle was no more infectious to primates than brain from scrapie-affected sheep. Certainly, the incubation period (time from injection to illness onset) was slightly longer for BSE than for scrapie.

What we had shown was that there was not an insurmountable 'species barrier' between cattle and primates. It was, therefore, not possible to argue

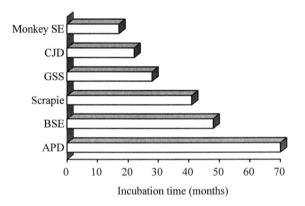

Fig. 8.2 Incubation times in a series of experimental transmissions of spongiform encephalopathy from different donor species to common marmosets. In each case the monkeys were injected intracerebrally (under anaesthetic) with the same volume of brain homogenate containing the same amount of brain taken from the donors at the end-stage of illness. The difference in incubation time is a measure of the species barrier. The transmission times for the human diseases (CJD and GSS) were much shorter than for the animal diseases (scrapie and BSE). Interestingly, the BSE transmissions took longer than the scrapie transmissions, suggesting that the BSE brain homogenates were no more infectious than the scrapie brain homogenates. The atypical prion disease (APD) case failed to transmit in 6 years. The donor was known to have died from prion disease because he carried the 144 bp insertion in the PrP gene and was a member of the pedigree illustrated elsewhere. The shortest incubation time is seen when monkey-adapted prion disease is transmitted to monkeys, that is, when there is no species barrier.

that BSE could not be transmitted to primates (including humans). Our experiments suggested that there was no specific reason to suppose that the BSE agent was more transmissible to primates than was the scrapie agent, for which the normal methods of consumption of sheep products did not appear to pose a risk to humans. What we did not address was the possibility that we might use sheep products differently from cattle products, for example, in the age of the animals from which meat was consumed, or the different tissues that are used from each species. Transmission of BSE to chimpanzees by the intracerebral route has not been attempted because, since the days of the first transmissions of CJD and kuru to chimpanzees, public opinion about the ethics of using chimpanzees for medical experiments has changed. Thus, it is not possible to determine whether transmission studies using monkeys would be appropriate for assessing the risk of BSE to humans. None the less, the European Commission has recommended that scientists should embark on large-scale experiments, planned to run for 10 years, to determine the minimum infectivity required to transmit BSE orally to monkeys, as a way of assessing whether BSE has caused CJD in humans. These plans also overlook 'the failure of all attempts to transmit CJD or kuru to susceptible non-human primates by the oral route, using huge infectious doses' (Masters *et al.* 1979).

This comment does not apply to *monkey-adapted* kuru or CJD, but the use of such tissue does address the issue of the species barrier between humans and non-humans. Either apes and monkeys are unlike humans in their susceptibility to these diseases or, and this is more likely to be the case, laboratory experiments using a small number of animals are unable to mimic what happens when a very large population is simultaneously exposed to a low level of infectivity.

Risk to man

It is actually quite difficult to assess minimum levels of risk. When a drug company develops a new treatment it will do a great deal of scientific research. It will use animals to assess whether the drug is likely to be toxic and cause unacceptable side-effects. A great many drugs are withdrawn at this stage and serious damage to humans is avoided. A drug that survives this assessment may then be prescribed to a limited number of named patients and, if all goes well, it will then be used on a known number of patients in a clinical trial. If, after all this, the drug appears to be safe, it can be released for general prescription. At this stage, when millions of pounds have been spent on drug development, a handful of patients out of perhaps hundreds of thousands of people who have been prescribed the drug may develop serious side-effects, and the drug will have to be withdrawn. Nothing can be done in terms of laboratory tests or limited clinical trials to prevent a drug having to be withdrawn at this very last stage. Similarly, any animal experiments designed to judge how dangerous the agent of BSE would be to humans cannot indicate that it will be so safe that not even a handful of cases of CJD will be caused in a population of 50 million people. If we knew that monkeys or chimpanzees were identical to humans in their sensitivity to the agent of BSE, and we were able to do studies in several hundred such animals, we would still be unable to make judgements about the safety of the human population. Even if we were to do the experiments in several hundred humans, we would not get meaningful results. It is quite likely that many thousands or even millions of people in Britain have eaten the same level of contamination which may have led to the new variant cases of CJD, and yet they have not become ill. Small-scale experiments in which animals do not get sick are likely to lead to false reassurance, and this could be extremely dangerous.

BSE has now been experimentally transmitted to a number of species, usually by intracerebral injection, including pigs, sheep, and goats, in addition to the mice mentioned above. All these transmissions have used brain tissue from BSE-affected animals as the source of the agent. Disease has never been transmitted by injecting tissue other than brain tissue. In other words, the transmissible agent of BSE has never been detected in any of the peripheral tissues of a 'naturally' infected cow. However, in a large experiment to investigate the development of infectivity and the pathological changes in cattle following the oral administration of a single dose of BSE-affected brain homogenate, Gerald Wells and his colleagues discovered that infectivity could be detected in the distal ileum (the end part of the intestine), 6 months after the dosing. Why this tissue should be infectious in 'laboratory' cases of BSE but not in 'field' cases remains a mystery. The whole of the intestinal system in cattle is included in Specified Bovine Offal. Incidentally, these scientists have shown that a calf fed a single dose of just 1 gram (about 1/30th of an ounce) of BSE brain homogenate can develop BSE. No prion disease has ever been proven to be transmissible between species by the oral route, using tissues other than brain and spinal cord.

The problem of the long time course

A major problem in studying BSE and the other prion diseases is the long time course over which these diseases develop. As we have seen, the incubation period from infecting event to illness onset can range from a few months in the case of mouse- and hamster-adapted scrapie models up to several years in larger animals, depending on the route of transmission. In humans, the incubation period can vary from 18 months in iatrogenic CJD to perhaps 40 years in kuru. Such time courses make the collection of epidemiological data, the identification of causative events, and experimental transmission studies (other than in rodents) difficult. The only direct way of measuring infectivity levels in various tissues is by experimental transmissions, and when this is done by injecting suspect tissue from one species (say a cow) into another (a mouse) the species barrier seriously reduces the sensitivity. Within-species transmission studies using large animals are made difficult by the relatively longer incubation periods in animals which live a long time, and they have only been carried out on a small scale. Thus it was that at the beginning of the BSE epidemic, when faced with a possible threat to public health, decisions had to be made without the benefit of information about the tissue distribution of infectivity in cattle, which would not be available for perhaps years. Mouse-adapted scrapie was considered too 'artificial' as a model, so scientists drew on the data from earlier experiments on sheep scrapie. There was a problem, however, in that the scrapie data were not collected in the expectation that major economic and public-health decisions would depend on them. As an example, the SBO Ban applied to tissues that had been found to be infectious in scrapie-affected sheep, but which have not subsequently been found to be infectious in BSE-affected cattle. If this ban proves to have been inadequate in protecting the public, it might be because the necessary tissues were not included in the ban, or because of a failure effectively to remove the tissues covered by the ban. It might, however, be because by spreading the ban too widely, to include non-infectious tissues, the efficiency with which the most infectious tissues (brain and spinal cord) is removed was compromised. Let us suppose, for example, that it is much more difficult to remove all the most infectious tissue than to remove most of the less infectious or non-infectious offals. (The amount of brain and spinal cord in an animal is much less than the amount of other specified offals, such as the intestines, spleen, etc.) Those responsible for removing the offals may feel satisfied if almost all of the specified offals are removed without appreciating that what is left is a substantial part of the most infectious brain and spinal cord. If the effort had been put into removing all the brain and spinal cord rather than large amounts of offal in which infectivity has never been detected, the ban might have been more effective. This is a common theme in safety procedures. It is always better to do exactly the right thing than to guess at what to do, even where that guess is thought to err on the safe side.

The public has not always appreciated that, since the incubation time of BSE in cattle is about 4–5 years, the course of the epidemic responds somewhat sluggishly to environmental events and to legislative measures to alter it. Although the changes in the rendering processes took place throughout the 1970s, the reduction in the use of solvents occurred at the beginning of the 1980s, leading to the view that effective exposure of cattle to infected feedstuff probably started in 1981/1982. The effects of an exposure which might have started as early as 1981 did not become apparent until the first cases of BSE in 1986. By the time Wilesmith's first epidemiological study was set up in mid-1987, some 50 000 cattle destined to die with BSE were already infected. It took a further 12 months to identify the feedstuff as the source of infection and to implement the Ruminant Feed Ban, during which time a further 35 000 animals, subsequently to get BSE, were infected. Of course, these figures refer to cattle living long enough to develop BSE, and do not include those infected animals which were killed, and probably eaten, before BSE claimed them.

BSE-affected animals born after the ban—the 'BABs'

The Ruminant Feed Ban was very effective in reducing the number of new infections. From 1984 to 1988, the numbers of animals born that were destined to get BSE rose steeply, but there was a dramatic fall in these births after the Ruminant Feed Ban was put in place. Of course the number of BSE cases continued to rise, reaching a peak at the end of 1992 and the beginning of 1993, after which the effects of the Ruminant Feed Ban began to be seen and the numbers of animals developing BSE began to fall. However, a substantial number of animals born after the Ruminant Feed Ban (known as BABs) have eventually succumbed to BSE. Those born shortly after the Ruminant Feed Ban, perhaps during the autumn or early winter of 1988, were probably infected with contaminated feedstuff which had been manufactured prior to the ban and which was still 'in the system'. The occurrence of BSE in animals born in 1989 has been attributed to 'leakage', that is to inadequate enforcement of, or compliance with, the regulations. Evidence for this was provided by Wilesmith's group, who examined the correlation between the incidence of BSE in BABs and the ratio of pigs and poultry to adult dairy cows in each county of England. This ingenious analysis showed that in areas where there were large numbers of pigs and poultry, relative to adult cows, there was also a higher incidence of BSE in BABs. Since the use of implicated meat-and-bone meal was still allowed in non-ruminant feedstuff, we might conclude that some of the pig feed was contaminating calf feedstuffs in the feed mills. A subsequent analysis of BSE in Northern Ireland confirms that the most likely explanation for the occurrence of BSE in BABs was that cross-contamination was occurring between pig feed and calf feed which was manufactured on the same premises (Denny and Hueston 1997). It is interesting to note that while the level of cross-contamination appears to have been sufficient to cause BSE in cows, the inclusion of large amounts of infectious material in pig feed has not resulted in any detectable disease in pigs. The SBO Ban (part 1), intended to prevent the use of specified bovine offals in human food, probably helped to reduce the leakage of SBOs into cattle feed by ensuring that more of it was destroyed, and leakage was reduced even further when the SBO Ban was extended (part 2) to prohibit the use of SBOs in all animal feedstuff, including that for pigs and poultry. Although a very small number of animals born in 1991 and later may be expected to develop BSE, the most recent epidemiological analysis suggests that new infections have virtually been eliminated. In the peak year of incidence, 1992, there were 36 681 confirmed cases of BSE. In 1995 there were 12 245 cases, which represents a decline in incidence from 0.92 per cent of all adult cattle to 0.33 per cent. Clearly, the Ruminant Feed Ban was an appropriate measure to control infection of cattle, but it took a further 3 years of legislation to ensure that the contaminated feedstuff was comprehensively excluded from the cattle diet. The epidemic may have been curtailed more quickly if, instead of banning the feeding of ruminant-derived protein to ruminants but leaving the option of feeding it to non-ruminants, the legislation had required that specified offals from cattle and sheep be totally destroyed. Most analysts think that BSE will disappear within the next few years, as long as there is no substantial maternal transmission. But more of that shortly.

Cats and kudu

Spongiform encephalopathy has also appeared as a new disease in a number of other animals. In May 1990, a group of veterinarians at Bristol University described a Siamese cat, Max, which, according to its owner, had started behaving oddly. It was the cat's pleasure to sleep on top of the television, but it had alarmed the owner by dropping off to sleep and then dropping off the television. Max had a spongiform encephalopathy. Before that time, SE had not been reported as a 'natural' disease of cats, although cats had been used successfully by Joe Gibbs and Carleton Gajdusek in experimental transmissions, so it was known that they were susceptible to prion disease. Over the following year or so, more cats developed the illness. These animals showed major signs of neurological dysfunction including ataxia (difficulty in organizing walking movements), particularly of the back legs, which led the animals to crouch when walking. In addition, the animals were, alternately, aggressive and timid. They tended to salivate excessively and, while some drank too much, others ate too much, suggesting that the brain control of these functions had been disturbed. The neurological signs seen in these animals were similar to those seen in cats injected intracerebrally with brain tissue from cases of Creutzfeldt–Jakob disease, and the Bristol scientists summarized their findings thus: 'The striking clinical and histopathological similarity of this disease to the previously described transmissible spongiform encephalopathies of animals, leaves little doubt about the nature of the disease' (Wyatt et al. 1991).

As is well known, sick cats often disappear and the cause of death is never established, and it is possible that an animal with a movement disorder would be more at risk of being run over when crossing the road. The Bristol University Veterinary School specializes in neurological diseases of cats, so, if this disease had not been a new disease, cases would almost certainly have turned up earlier in Bristol. By the beginning of 1997, the total number of cases of feline spongiform encephalopathy (FSE) was about 70. It is assumed that the cats acquired FSE as a result of consuming contaminated cat food, and the likely culprit was the pelleted feedstuff which, like the cattle feedstuff, contained ruminant-derived meat-and-bone meal. Interestingly, one cat in Liechtenstein and another in Norway have developed FSE. The source of infection in these particular cats is not known, although the animal in Liechtenstein was born and lived close to the area in Switzerland that had had more than 200 cases of BSE at that time. So far no dogs have developed SE, even though some of the dry dog food and biscuits contained the same meat-and-bone meal. The reason for this remains a mystery. Reports of spongiform encephalopathies in other species appeared throughout the late 1980s up to the mid-1990s, usually as a single case report and then, when a number of animals of the same species had developed the disease, as a general account of the clinical and neuropathological picture for that species. Eventually, as further cases in the same species appeared, these were not published in the scientific literature, although veterinary epidemiologists and officials at MAFF kept a close tally on numbers. In addition to the domestic cats, a few large zoo cats have developed SE, including three cheetahs, a puma, an ocelot, and a tiger. Such zoo cats are usually fed meat which may have come from animal knackers and could have included cows with BSE.

Epidemiological studies of BSE have provided no evidence of horizontal transmission, that is of disease being passed directly from one animal to another. But an outbreak of spongiform encephalopathy in the herd of greater kudu at London Zoo raised the spectre of horizontal transmission. Spongiform encephalopathy had already appeared in a number of larger antelopes (described in the scientific literature as 'exotic ungulates'), such as the nyala, eland, gemsbok, and Arabian oryx. London Zoo has kept a small herd of greater kudu since 1970. As we have come to expect by now, the clinical signs in these animals consisted of ataxia, although, because of the rapid progression of disease, the animals had to be killed within a few days of onset. This extremely fast course of disease has also been seen in spongiform encephalopathy in other exotic ungulates and in a few cases of BSE in cattle and scrapie in sheep. Indeed, one of the monkeys to which BSE was transmitted experimentally appeared perfectly healthy in the morning (remember this was some 4 years after the animals had been injected) but within a few hours had developed neurological signs serious enough to be considered life-threatening later the same afternoon.

Like most grazing animals kept in captivity, kudu had been fed supplements containing added protein in the form of meat-and-bone meal, but only up until 1987. Eight of these graceful creatures were born between 1987 and 1993 and, of these, five (Linda, Karla, Kas, Bambi, and the prosaically named 346/90) developed spongiform encephalopathy. In a paper describing this miniature epidemic, one of the zoo's veterinarians reported that, with the possible exception of the first case, none of the animals was knowingly fed feedstuff containing meat-and-bone-meal (Kirkwood et al. 1993).

This outbreak raised certain important issues. First, the proportion of affected animals was higher than that seen even in those herds of cattle most badly affected with BSE and, secondly, the pattern of disease incidence suggested that cases were not exclusively linked to consumption of feedstuffs containing ruminant-derived protein. The investigators thought it likely that the BSE agent entered the herd in contaminated feedstuff around 1987, but that subsequently the disease was transmitted directly from animal to animal. They were unable to suggest a possible mode of transmission since transmissible agent has not been detected in faeces, urine, milk, or saliva in scrapie or BSE, so horizontal transmission must be regarded as speculation. However, feedstuffs containing meat-and-bone meal were fed to other species on the premises and it is possible that the kudu were inadvertently fed this material. One female was the mother or grandmother to all the affected animals, so a genetic involvement or susceptibility cannot be ruled out and this might account for the high proportion of affected animals. Spongiform encephalopathy in a kudu and her daughter led at first to suspicions of maternal transmission, but the subsequent appearance of spongiform encephalo-pathy in the other kudu which were not the direct progeny of affected animals, as well as in five other exotic ungulates born in several zoos in Britain, suggests that a more widespread source of infection was responsible. All of these other exotic ungulates had unaffected dams and were born either before the Ruminant Feed Ban of 1988, or between that ban and the more stringent Specified Offals Ban of 1989. No other cases have occurred since 1992. The animals born between 1988 and 1990 could have been infected by the supposed widespread, but low-level, contamination of many types of animal feed, which the Specified Offals Ban seems to have largely eliminated.

Beware the ides of March

The middle of March 1996 was a frenetic time for the SEAC Committee as they deliberated the meaning of the most recent findings of the CJD Surveillance Unit. On 19 March 1996, the SEAC Committee reported to Mr Stephen Dorrell, the then Health Secretary, who announced in Parliament the following day that 10 cases of a new variant of CJD had been detected in young people in Britain in the previous 2 years, and that the most likely explanation at that time was that 'these cases are linked to BSE before the introduction of the SBO [Specified Bovine Offals] Ban of 1989'. On 20 March 1996, the 'Farming Today' programme on BBC Radio 4 warned that the beef industry was about to collapse. By lunch time, it had. Beef consumption in

Britain had been in slow decline for many years before BSE was known about, partly because beef was becoming expensive relative to chicken and pork, and partly because more meat was being sold pre-cooked, with many of these convenience foods using chicken rather than beef. Increasing awareness of BSE may have contributed to this decline, but only the announcement that BSE had probably caused disease in cats had had an abrupt effect from which the industry took some time to recover. Now it was different. Beef sales in Britain dropped dramatically. What had not been expected was the violent reaction of the Europeans. Beef sales on the continent dropped much more than in Britain, and remain deeply depressed. The European Commission (EC) banned the exportation of any bovine product from Britain to anywhere in the world (so that it could not be brought back into Europe by the back door). Rather than placating the European population and persuading them to resume eating continental beef, the very seriousness of the EC's measures seemed to put Europeans off beef completely. After all, how could they be really sure where it had come from? Indeed, there have been reports of British beef entering continental Europe illegally.

With considerable speed the Government introduced the '30 Month Scheme' in Britain. This banned the inclusion of any part of a cow aged over 30 months in human food. This can be regarded as act of genius or of madness depending on your perspective. The Government believed public health to be adequately protected by the SBO Ban of 1989, but reckoned that the public would not be able to cope with the implications of the long incubation times in cattle or people, and would want something done *now*. People also expected their milk to be available as usual. The milking of dairy cows was allowed until they were no longer economically viable, but then they had to be destroyed rather than eaten. The prime beef industry (where cases of BSE had been rare) was partially protected because the best quality beef is usually taken from cattle just under 30 months old, so there would be plenty of meat in the shops. Cattle under 30 months old were born after 1993, at a time at which it had been calculated that the Ruminant Feed Ban had been totally effective. So the last cows destined to get BSE were already over 30 months old and the public could be assured that the meat they were eating was BSE-free. There was, however, a darker side to this legislation. The owners of pedigree herds, who they had spent a lifetime building up breeding stock, were frequently ruined. Many abattoirs closed instantly either because they had no cattle to process for food or because they were unable to comply with regulations concerning the disposal of cattle not destined for consumption. The disposal of carcasses was a gruesome problem. Burning would have created excessive smoke pollution.

Burial was impracticable and unsafe. Burial does not destroy the agent, so large numbers of hidden cattle dumps could have been a hazard in the future. Condemned cattle could not be rendered in plants that were used for the rendering of any material that was to be used for feeding any farm animal. Rendered material still had to be destroyed and large amounts of storage space had to be found until adequate incineration could be arranged. Thousands of carcasses were held in frozen storage, producing a 'meat iceberg', while people discussed how to dispose of them. A queue of dairy cows awaiting slaughter grew daily throughout the summer of 1996, and farmers were very concerned at the prospect of buying expensive feedstuff (which was by now in short supply) to keep these animals alive over the coming winter. It took until the end of the year to clear the backlog of cattle and to get the disposal of carcasses running fairly smoothly. Compensation was paid for cattle covered by the scheme, but any perturbation in a complex and finely balanced industry, together with all its subsidiary industries (where compensation was often not paid), leads to many bankruptcies and redundancies. Even when a crisis is sorted out fairly quickly, jobs may be lost forever.

The ban on exports of all cattle, including calves, to Europe put an abrupt end to a political protest that had been disrupting ports in southern England in the summer of 1996. Cows only produce milk after they have had a calf. Consequently, the dairy industry produces an excess of calves, most of which are eaten as veal. Veal is not popular in Britain, partly because of worries over the welfare of the animals (although this does not stop people drinking the milk that generates the surplus of calves), so most of these veal calves were exported to the continent. The political protest was about the conditions in which these calves were kept on the continent, and particularly during transport. The BSE crisis put a complete stop to the export of veal calves. Many of them were just killed instead. It was anticipated that by the end of 1997 there would be a shortage of young cattle to supply the dairy industry and that cattle would have to be imported from continental Europe. Since surveillance of BSE is less stringent in continental Europe, this opens up the possibility that just as the BSE epidemic draws to a close in the UK, BSE-infected animals will find their way into the country.

Europe

The reason why the BSE epidemic occurred in Britain and not elsewhere is difficult to answer because the precise cause of the onset of the epidemic is not known. If BSE came from sheep scrapie, the fact that Britain had more scrapie than the rest of Europe may be relevant. Although changes in the rendering system probably made a contribution to the spread of BSE, it has not been established that the pre-1980 methods of rendering definitely did destroy the scrapie agent. Furthermore, the rendering practices employed in continental Europe were not so different from those used in Britain, although both have been changed in the light of the epidemic. During the first half of the 1980s, when as many as 50 000 cows in Britain may have become infected with BSE before the first cases of illness were diagnosed, many thousands of tons of rendered material were exported to Europe for many purposes, including the feeding of cattle. After the Ruminant Feed Ban of 1988 the surplus rendered (and contaminated) material was legally exported to the continent (Butler 1996). There were many uses for rendered protein and it was up to the recipient countries to make their own internal regulations. In addition, many calves were exported to the continent and, while most of them were eaten as veal, some entered the adult herd as milkers or breeding stock. Many European countries have reported the occurrence of a few cases of BSE in cattle imported from Britain, but there has been no general recognition of a BSE epidemic occurring in cattle born in continental Europe, except for some cases in Switzerland. Some countries have instituted the equivalent of a Ruminant Feed Ban and an SBO Ban; others have not. Some countries have an efficient BSE monitoring scheme; others do not. Any country that has even a very low level of BSE, and which does not have an effective Ruminant Feed Ban, is likely to have a major epidemic of BSE in the future and, if the new variant of CJD is caused by eating contaminated beef products, any country that has any BSE and does not have an effective SBO Ban is putting its people at risk. Any country that does not know whether it has BSE or not is potentially in trouble. Where BSE exists without adequate protection of its cattle to prevent recycling, there is likely to be a major epidemic at any time in the next 15 years. Britain may have made a lot of mistakes the first time round, but the same mistakes do not have to be made again.

The eradication of BSE

Despite the fact that the '30 Month Scheme' prevented the consumption of any meat from a cow that was incubating BSE, there was a demand from the British public and from the Europeans for the eradication of all cases of BSE. It was clear that so long as cases of BSE were being found in Britain, the EC would not lift its ban on the export of British beef or bovine products. The only thing to do was to kill all the cows that might be going to get BSE. In August 1996, a paper appeared in the journal *Nature*, which presented a detailed mathematical model of the BSE epidemic up to the previous month (Anderson *et al.* 1996). As of July 1996 the total number of confirmed cases of BSE stood at 161 412 and the authors calculated that about 7000 more animals would develop BSE before the epidemic was over, by the year 2000 or 2001. Most of the paper was devoted to culling strategies and presented a series of cost–benefit schemes to eliminate those remaining animals destined to get BSE. Of course, all the 7000 animals would be eliminated if all 9 360 000 cattle in the UK were killed immediately, but this would mean that 1300 healthy cattle would be killed for each case of BSE prevented. It was also not practicable because killing and disposing of the carcasses of so many cows would have taken many months, and most of the cows destined to get BSE would have done so while waiting their turn for slaughter. The most efficient culling policy, according to the authors, would be to slaughter all birth cohorts (that is, all calves born on the same farm during the same calving season as a case of BSE) plus the offspring of BSE-affected cows. This approach, they calculated, would prevent about 1500 of the 7000 cases at a cost of some 44 000 animals. The reader will observe that this culling strategy assumes that some of the animals yet to get BSE will do so as a result of maternal transmission from its dam. Does maternal transmission of BSE really occur?

The answer is 42. But what was the question?

In Douglas Adams's *The hitch hiker's guide to the galaxy* (Adams 1979), a mixture of witty comedy and science fiction, Mr Arthur Dent and his mentor, Ford Prefect, attempt to answer the Ultimate Question of Life, the Universe, and Everything. Their computer, Deep Thought, spent seven and a half million years calculating the answer, which turned out to be 42.

'I checked it very thoroughly,' said the computer, 'and that quite definitely is the answer. I think the problem, to be quite honest with you, is that you've never actually known what the question is.'

In 1989, an experiment was set up by MAFF and the Central Veterinary Laboratory to address the question of whether or not maternal transmission of BSE occurred. By maternal transmission of disease we mean the passing on of disease from a mother to its offspring either prenatally (by way of the placenta), during the birth process, or postnatally (by some process specific to the mother–offspring relationship, such as suckling or licking clean). Calves were purchased from BSE-affected herds and consisted of one or more pairs of animals, of which one member of the pair was the calf of a cow which subsequently developed BSE (BSE+ve dam), while the other was a calf of the same age from a cow that had reached 6 years of age without developing BSE (BSE-ve dam). A total of 315 such pairs of animals, which ranged in age from a few months to about 18 months, were collected and housed on a number of experimental husbandry farms run by MAFF. All the calves were to be observed for a total of 7 years to see whether the offspring of BSE+ve dams were any more likely to develop BSE than the offspring of the BSE-ve dams. (If a BSE-ve dam later developed BSE, both animals in the pair were removed from the study.)

This study was nearing completion, with the youngest animal due to be 7 years old in November 1996, when Mr Dorrell's announcement came in March of that year. A great deal of pressure was put on the investigators directing the maternal transmission experiments to publish the results so far. The experiment had been carried out 'blind', with those who were assessing whether or not calves were showing signs of BSE being unaware of the BSE status of the mother. 'Blind' studies are designed to prevent the judgement of investigators being influenced by knowledge of the group to which each subject belongs. The investigators were reluctant to 'break the code' before the experiment was completed, but eventually released the data when 273 pairs of calves had reached 7 years of age. Thirteen of the offspring of the BSE-ve dams and 42 of the offspring of the BSE+ve dams had developed BSE. The difference was immediately interpreted as evidence for maternal transmission. But was maternal transmission the best explanation for the excess? Was the right question being asked?

A number of possible explanations for the excess come to mind: a selection bias in the way these calves were collected; genetic susceptibility to infection with the agent of BSE; and maternal transmission of the agent from the incubating (but not overtly sick) dam to the offspring. The raw data (42 versus 13) cannot differentiate between genetic susceptibility and maternal transmission. So why was maternal transmission assumed? The answer probably lies in the widespread belief that scrapie disease in sheep is maternally transmitted, a belief based on work published in the 1960s and 1970s. In this early work it was shown that the best predictor of whether or not a lamb would contract scrapie was the scrapie status of its mother. The scrapie status of the father was not usually known since a ram was often brought in to serve, or tup, a large flock of ewes and then returned or sold on. However, as we described earlier, we recently re-analysed the early data claiming to provide evidence for maternal transmission of scrapie disease in sheep, and concluded that the data could not support the claim. We found that the original data showed no deviation from genetic inheritance of scrapie. We also stressed the fact that there is no evidence for maternal transmission of disease in any of the human spongiform encephalopathies, including kuru, which reached high prevalence levels in Papua New Guinea in the 1950s (Ridley and Baker 1995). Furthermore, Nora Hunter and her colleagues at the Neuropathogenesis Unit in Edinburgh have analysed disease occurrence in a flock of sheep specially bred to be susceptible to scrapie infection. In their studies of the genetic basis of this susceptibility, they concluded that there was no evidence of maternal transmission of scrapie from ewe to lamb (Hunter *et al.* 1996). This conclusion is important since scientists at this unit have generally supported the case for maternal transmission. Moreover, there is no established mechanism by which maternal transmission would occur. Data on infectivity in blood and placenta in sheep are inadequate and, as we have seen, experiments have failed to detect infectivity in milk or any tissue other than brain and spinal cord in field cases of BSE.

There is another way of looking at the data. If the difference in BSE levels between the offspring of BSE+ve and BSE-ve dams was the result of a difference in genetic susceptibility to contamination from feedstuff, rather than a reflection of direct maternal transmission of disease, this difference should become smaller as the contaminated feedstuff is removed. Some of the pairs of calves collected for this experiment were born before the 1988 Ruminant Feed Ban, although most were born afterwards. Those born before the Ruminant Feed Ban would have had a higher exposure to contaminated material than those born after the ban. If the data from the experiment are looked at separately for those born before the ban and those born after the ban, we find that the difference between the offspring of BSE+ve dams and BSE-ve dams is markedly reduced in those born after the ban. We would have expected the degree to which an infected mother could transmit disease directly to her offspring would be independent of the Ruminant Feed Ban, but it does seem that this is not the case. In other words, we think a better interpretation of these data is that the BSE+ve dams contracted disease because they were susceptible to the contaminated feedstuff, and that they passed this genetic susceptibility on to their calves. The BSE-ve dams were likely to be somewhat resistant to disease since they had lived through the main part of the BSE epidemic without developing BSE, and they would have passed this genetic resistance on to their calves.

Any genetic difference in susceptibility to the infectious agent in the feedstuff would have been more apparent in calves born before the Ruminant Feed Ban, when the higher exposure would have selected out the susceptible calves. If what was being passed on to the calves from the BSE+ve cows was the agent itself, this effect would have been more marked in the calves born after the Ruminant Feed Ban when fewer of the control animals would have acquired BSE from the residual contamination in the feedstuff. It might have been appropriate if the investigators had asked the question, 'Will this experiment be able to distinguish between maternal transmission and genetic susceptibility?' (Ridley and Baker 1996a.)

The code of the maternal transmission experiment had been broken in response to public concern during the summer of 1996. The final details of this experiment were available at the end of January 1997, when the brains of the last cow to die had been processed. The number of pairs of animals completing the experiment was 301, since some pairs had had to be withdrawn for technical reasons. The answer remains 42, but the SEAC Committee accepts that the experimental design could not distinguish between maternal transmission and genetic susceptibility.

Public attitudes

The general public in Britain and in parts of continental Europe has been more exercised over the possibility of BSE posing a risk to humans than over any other 'food scare' in recent times, although the concern did not seem to increase greatly after March 1996. Various factors can be identified that contribute to the public perception of risk, and many of those features known to contribute to an increase in concern can be seen to apply to BSE. First, people generally underestimate high risks and overestimate low risks; in some cases two such contrasted risks may change places in peoples' perceptions. For example, the risk of being killed while flying is less in terms of miles travelled than the risk of being killed on the roads, but many people experience more anxiety before a flight than they do before getting into a car. Suggestions that the risk posed to humans by BSE was 'remote' or 'extremely small' may have generated more anxiety before March 1996 than the suggestion made at that time that, based on the events of the previous 2 years, the risk then stood at about 5 cases per 50 million people per year.

People also like to feel that they have control over the risks that they choose to take. For example, they may tolerate a high risk in a dangerous sport because they choose to participate but be much less tolerant of a risk that they feel has been imposed on them from outside. Indeed, people seem to have a kind of 'risk thermostat', which determines the degree of risk that they are happy to live with; imposing a degree of risk on them deprives them of the choice of 'spending' some of their risk-tolerance on something they like. Individuals are particularly prone to feel that they have little control over risks for which the source or mechanism is poorly understood, which cannot be constantly monitored, and which may affect an unspecified and, therefore potentially large, number of people. BSE fulfils all these criteria.

Food researchers have found that very many people have an over-optimistic view of their diet. The majority of those questioned seem to believe that their own diet is more healthy than average, which logically cannot be true. Most people believe that they have reduced their fat intake in the past 10 years, whereas sales indicate that fat consumption by the nation as a whole has not gone down. In our own experience, most people that we have asked claim either that they do not eat beef or that their consumption of beef and beef products has been reduced as a result of the BSE scare and, while national consumption has gone down somewhat, sales are much less depressed than these answers would suggest. This is, of course, not a controlled sample; their social class is not representative of the country, and they may be unaware of quite how much beef product is incorporated in unrecognizable form into processed food.

The government announcement in March 1996, that several cases of CJD in young people in Britain might be BSE-related, resulted in a short-lived period of extreme concern in the general public followed, paradoxically, by relative calm. It seemed that the public coped better with a risk that was real, but which was perceived as small, rather than with the previous uncertainty. As an editorial in the *Lancet* pointed out, there was no way of knowing at that time whether BSE would result in the death of no one (that is, the new variant of CJD is not BSE-related), or several million people over the course of 40 years. It may take several years before precise predictions can be made (*Lancet* 1996).

9

New variant CJD, a disease of old age in young people

Crisis day

The announcement by the Secretary of State for Health in March 1996 that a new form of CJD had been discovered which could be related to BSE had an immediate impact on the public perception of the risks posed by the BSE epidemic. The news was shocking, but on what was it based? Given the wide range of presentations of CJD in individual cases, what could constitute a new variant of CJD? How could it be related to BSE? The Secretary of State had been careful to say only that 'the most likely explanation' of these cases was that they were related to BSE. How could he be sure that the exposure had occurred before 1989? He was acting on the advice of the Spongiform Encephalopathy Advisory Committee (SEAC), which, it emerged, had been in conference for the previous few days. The SEAC Committee was convinced that the accumulated number of cases of CJD in young people over the previous 2 years was sufficient to indicate that these cases had an unusual origin. So just what was the evidence that they were likely to be BSE-related?

Incidence of CJD in Britain

When the CJD Surveillance Unit was set up in 1990, its brief had been to monitor CJD in Britain, and to determine whether there was an increase in the number of cases which might suggest that BSE was a risk to human health. Implicit was the supposition that, if BSE caused disease in people, that disease would look like CJD. From 1980 to 1990 the number of cases of

CJD diagnosed each year in Great Britain was about 25. When the CJD Surveillance Unit began looking intensively, the number of cases rose steadily to about 40 per year. Most of this increase could be accounted for by the additional number of very elderly people who received a diagnosis of CJD. It is easy to see that, without an active surveillance system, very elderly patients who had a slowly progressive form of CJD might be thought to have Alzheimer's disease (which is very common in the elderly), while patients who had very rapid onset CJD might be thought to have had a stroke, or some other geriatric condition. Even this higher number of cases was not greatly different from that found in the rest of Europe, where the incidence of CJD had also been rising because of more precise diagnostic methods. No one had been surprised that the hard work of the CJD Surveillance Unit had found a few more cases of CJD. In addition, the number of cases varied quite a bit from one year to another, so the occurrence of an extra five cases in each of the previous 2 years (1994 and 1995) was not sufficient, in numerical terms, to warrant concern. Something else was different about these patients.

The occurrence of the new cases

The first 10 cases of the new variant of CJD (nvCJD) were described in a paper by Bob Will and colleagues in the *Lancet*, in April 1996 (Will *et al.* 1996). The four men and six women had become ill between February 1994 and October 1995. Detailed information was available about the previous life and habits of nine of the patients. None had had neurosurgery or received human pituitary-derived growth hormone, so they had not acquired CJD through any of the known iatrogenic routes. Four patients had never had any general surgical operation, two had had their tonsils removed, one had had an operation on her foot, and one had had a minor gynaecological procedure. The ninth patient had a complicated medical history involving several operations, but, since she was the only patient in the group to have undergone any major surgery, it seemed unlikely that these patients had acquired CJD from some previously unsuspected but plausible medical intervention.

The patients did not appear to have had any exceptional exposure to BSE-affected cattle. One had worked as a butcher for a couple of years at the very beginning of the BSE epidemic, and another had visited an abbatoir in 1987, but this hardly counts as exceptional exposure. None of them had ever worked on farms, although one had taken regular holidays on a dairy farm before 1986. All nine patients for whom data were available had eaten beef and beef products, but none had had an exceptional diet, and one had been a vegetarian since 1991. There really was nothing special about this group of people to suggest why they, in particular, should have become affected with this new variant of CJD. Although three of the patients had already been reported in the literature as being unusual presentations of CJD, a connection with BSE had not been made at that time (Bateman *et al.* 1995; Britton *et al.* 1995; Howard 1996).

Age at onset

Eight of the patients had died between the ages of 19 and 41 years. Two patients were still alive when the first report of the new variant of CJD was published. They were 18 and 31 years old at that time. The ages at onset ranged from 16 to 39 years. This was deeply worrying. The peak age at onset for sporadic CJD lies between 60 and 70 years of age, although the age-related incidence begins to rise from 35 years upwards. In Britain, only four cases of CJD had occurred in people under 35 years old in the 20 years between 1970 and the end of 1989. Now four cases in 1994 and five cases in 1995 had had an onset at less than 35 years. Of the 10 cases of nvCJD, six were younger even than 30 years, whereas only four cases of CJD under 30 years had ever previously been reported anywhere in the world. Even taking into account the overall rise in the number of cases detected in Britain in the past few years, six such young cases in 2 years seemed too many.

Even though the age at onset had been the main factor in alerting the CJD Surveillance Unit to the occurrence of a new form of CJD, there was little reason to expect that, if BSE led to CJD, it would be mainly in young people. Indeed, if the incubation period was many years long the disease would not occur in very young children. Although children might be more likely to 'catch' conventional infectious diseases such as measles or chickenpox this is because most adults have developed immunity to these common diseases. But adults are not protected from prion disease by their immune systems. The immune system does not mount a conventional attack on the infectious agent in prion disease. This is further evidence that the agent is made only of host-coded protein and is therefore regarded as 'self' and not 'foreign' by the body's immune system.

The long incubation periods found in cases of prion disease, where the contaminating event can be determined (for example, in the growth hormone cases and in some of the kuru cases), might suggest that BSE-related disease would occur in people who were older rather than younger than average. This has sometimes led to the rather cavalier suggestion (made by adults) that children should be protected from BSE, because, if they did become infected, they would die in adulthood, whereas adults could happily go on eating the beef they enjoyed because they were likely to die from something else before the incubation period was over. It has been a much repeated story that the incubation period in kuru was always in excess of 20 or 30 years. In fact the incubation period in kuru ranged from about 3 years to over 30 years. It has also been argued that the late age at onset in sporadic CJD reflects an incubation period in excess of 40 years following exposure to an infectious agent, probably in infancy. We believe this argument to be wrong since we think that sporadic CJD is not acquired from an external source of infection at all.

The occurrence of nvCJD in young people was, however, very unexpected, even though this was one of the main reasons for recognizing it as being different from sporadic CJD, and it is possible that, with time, the age range of nvCJD will extend to cover older people, assuming, of course, that it is BSE-related. New variant CJD will, however, be found in even younger people only if the minimum incubation period is less than 10 years, and if there was continuing contamination of human food after the Specified Offals Ban in 1989. If cases of nvCJD in Britain have been missed (that is, received a different, inaccurate diagnosis), they are likely to have been in older people, since there are more alternative neurological diseases with an older age at onset with which such cases could be confused.

Clinical symptoms

The clinical picture of the new variant form of CJD differed from that seen in sporadic CJD. Was this because nvCJD was acquired from an environmental source of contamination such as BSE-infected meat products, or was it because this is what sporadic CJD looked like in a young person? Nine of the 10 cases of nvCJD had been referred to a psychiatrist rather than a neurologist in the first instance, although this may reflect cultural perceptions of the cause of illness in young people, rather than a clear absence of neurological signs in the early stages of the disease. Several patients had exhibited personality change, behavioural abnormality, or depression, which would be considered in the first instance to have a psychiatric origin. Two patients had problems with their memory, but this could have been for psychiatric or neurological reasons. Two other patients had pains and discomfort in their limbs as very early symptoms. At this point it would have been impossible to make a positive diagnosis, but, as the illness progressed, they all developed ataxia (difficulty in co-ordinating and executing movements). Except in people who are drunk (in whom the brain is only temporarily not working properly), this sort of movement disorder is a sure sign of serious brain damage. A short time afterwards, the patients showed intellectual deterioration which eventually developed into a profound dementia. It would have been clear by the time of the onset of ataxia that these patients were suffering from a very serious neurological disease. The development of ataxia before dementia is unusual in sporadic CJD. Seven of the nvCJD cases developed myoclonus, that is, involuntary muscle spasms which, in combination with ataxia and dementia, is a good indicator of CJD. None of the patients with nvCJD had the particular pattern of EEG (electroencephalogram, the measurement of electrical activity in the brain by recording from electrodes placed on the scalp) that is highly characteristic of sporadic CJD. The clinical symptoms in these patients were, therefore, sufficiently like those of sporadic CJD to bring these cases to the attention of the CJD Surveillance Unit, but sufficiently different to indicate that they did not have sporadic CJD as it was then defined.

Comparison of cases of nvCJD with young-onset cases of CJD

Although sporadic CJD has a later average age at onset than nvCJD, CJD caused by contaminated growth hormone (ghCJD) usually occurred in young adults, because they were injected with growth hormone as children and the incubation period was from 5 to 25 years. So nvCJD cases could be compared to ghCJD cases which had a similar age at onset. New variant CJD and ghCJD differed in certain important ways. Like nvCJD, the majority of ghCJD cases presented with ataxia as an early symptom, with dementia appearing later in the disease, and the EEG characteristic of sporadic CJD was absent in both nvCJD and ghCJD. Could the nvCJD cases have received growth hormone treatment? This was most unlikely since that treatment programme was very specialized, all the patients were known, and none of the nvCJD cases had had an illness which would have warranted such a treatment. There is a 'black market' in growth hormone which has been taken illegally as a growth promoter by a small number of athletes, but there was no reason to think that the nvCJD cases were involved in any such practice. As we shall see in the next section, nvCJD and ghCJD resemble each other to some extent in their neuropathology, but they also differ sufficiently to suggest that they have different origins. That nvCJD and ghCJD resemble each other because they are both caused by contamination with infectious agent from an external source via the peripheral part of the body (intramuscular injections for ghCJD and the oral route for nvCJD) is plausible, but conjectural.

Florid plaques

Two nvCJD cases had undergone a brain biopsy procedure in which a small piece of brain was surgically removed, under anaesthetic, and examined under the microscope. In the remaining cases the brains were examined after death. All 10 cases showed spongiform change sufficient to give an unequivocal diagnosis of CJD. This spongiform change was present throughout the thalamus and basal ganglia (two very large parts of the brain around which the outer cortex is wrapped). There were also patches of spongiform change throughout the cortex (the outer part of the brain) and the cerebellum (a rather separate structure at the back of the brain concerned with movement and balance). The most outstanding feature of the neuropathology in all 10 cases, however, was the massive number of plaques spread throughout the brain. These plaques contained prion protein (PrP) as revealed by immunohistochemical staining. They resembled most closely the plaques seen in the brains of the majority of patients with kuru. (Large numbers of kuru-affected brain sections are stored in neuropathological archives.) So, again, these cases looked like other acquired cases of CJD, and less like sporadic CJD where only about 10–15 per cent have any plaques. The plaques in the brains of the nvCJD cases also had a special feature. The round deposit of PrP, which formed the middle of the plaques, was surrounded by a particularly large number of spongy vacuoles, giving it the appearance of a flower with a halo of petals. The term 'florid' was coined to describe this particular type of plaque. Florid plaques had never been seen in human brain before and, together with the unusual clinical symptoms, became part of the definitive description of nvCJD.

Some months after the first report of nvCJD was published, an important paper appeared reporting the results of a detailed examination of the brains of three macaque monkeys to which BSE had been experimentally transmitted some time before (using intracerebral injection of brain tissue from a BSE-affected cow). In addition to spongiform change, these monkeys

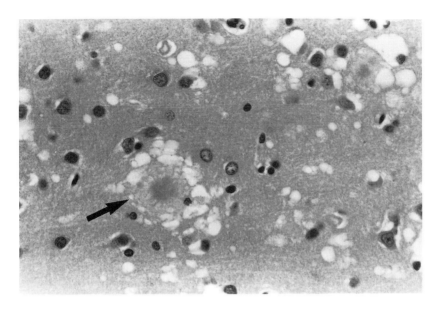

Fig. 9.1 A section from the brain of a patient with new variant CJD, showing a characteristically 'florid' plaque, consisting of a central core of PrP-amyloid surrounded by a ring of spongy vacuoles (magnification ∼ 400; photograph by J. W. Ironside).

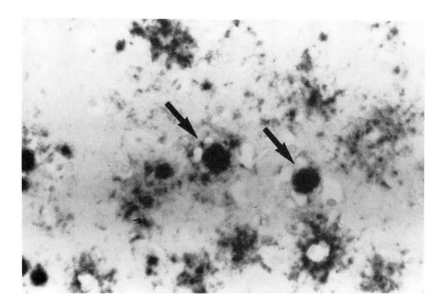

Fig. 9.2 A section from the brain of a patient with new variant CJD, which has been stained with an antibody to reveal the prion protein in the dark central core of a 'florid' plaque (magnification ∼ 400; photograph by J. W. Ironside).

had florid plaques (Lasmézas *et al.* 1996). So was there a link between florid plaques and BSE, and was the occurrence of florid plaques in the nvCJD cases sufficient evidence to link nvCJD with BSE? Possibly, but it was not quite that simple. The brains of cows with BSE and other animals, such as cats, which had been inadvertently infected with BSE do not have florid plaques. However, North American mule deer with chronic wasting disease (a prion disease of totally obscure origin) do have florid plaques. Plaques of varying degrees of 'floridness' can be found in certain forms of scrapie in sheep. Marmosets infected with BSE have plaque-like PrP deposits, but these are not identical to florid plaques, while marmosets infected with scrapie have fewer of these plaque-like deposits. So, while the occurrence of many florid plaques in humans may be sufficient to produce a diagnosis of nvCJD, the occurrence of florid plaques tells us little about how such cases are related to prion disease in other species, and do not prove that nvCJD is BSE-related.

Plaques and genes

The first 10 cases of nvCJD all had methionine at codon 129 on both copies of their PrP genes. In other words, they were codon 129 methionine homozygous. This could be a chance observation since 37 per cent of the British population is homozygous for methionine. However, it could indicate that, as for sporadic and iatrogenic CJD, people who are heterozygous at codon 129 (that is they carry one methionine and one valine) are partially protected from this form of CJD. Since only 11 per cent of the British population is homozygous for valine at codon 129, it is possible that there just has not been a case of nvCJD in such a person yet. It might really be the case, however, that only people who are homozygous for methionine at codon 129 are susceptible to nvCJD. This may come as some reassurance to a proportion of the population (though less so for the rest), but it is too soon to be sure what will happen in the long term.

That the first cases of nvCJD all had PrP plaques was somewhat surprising because in sporadic CJD such plaques are only seen in patients who have at least one valine at codon 129, and the nvCJD cases were all methionine homozygous. This striking difference strongly suggests that the cause of nvCJD is very different from the cause of sporadic CJD. However, all cases of ghCJD have plaques (though not florid plaques), irrespective of whether they carry methionine 129 or valine 129 (Ironside 1996*b*). This comparison with ghCJD is important because it raises the awful question of whether nvCJD could be related to some contamination of food or medicine in Britain which is unconnected with BSE. The question is awful because if it is true, it will not be possible to get rid of this source of contamination until it is found, and the ruination of the beef industry will all have been in vain. Nothing is known about the first 10 cases of nvCJD that makes them in any way medically exceptional before their illness. As a group they had not received any unusual medicine or other treatment. It is very difficult to think of any conceivable source of contamination from human or animal products, but it is worth considering the possibility, lest our obsession with BSE should blind us to another tragedy.

A case in France

At the time of its first description, the only reason for linking nvCJD to BSE was that all the cases had occurred in Britain about 10 years after the beginning of the BSE epidemic, under circumstances where an incubation period of several years might have been anticipated. This link would be weakened if more cases of nvCJD were to be found outside the UK. Shortly after nvCJD was first identified, a case was reported in France (Chazot *et al.* 1996). This 26-year-old patient had an illness very similar to that of the British nvCJD cases, and the neuropathology looked identical. So had this man eaten contaminated beef of British origin, or eaten contaminated beef from continental Europe, suggesting perhaps that there were more cases of BSE on the continent than had previously been recognized, or did this case indicate that nvCJD was not in fact BSE-related? The patient had not visited Britain; indeed his only foreign travel had been a short visit to Spain.

British beef products have, of course, been exported to France and many other countries, and this could have been the source of the risk to this French patient. The number of recorded cases of BSE in France was less than 20 up to 1996. It seems unlikely that such a small number could have caused a case of nvCJD if 160 000 confirmed cases of BSE in Britain had led, by 1996, to only 10 cases of nvCJD in Britain. There are those who have argued that, bearing in mind the vast amount of rendered meat and bone meal legally exported to France during the late 1980s, and the number of calves exported to France, not all of which were eaten as veal, there must have been more cases of BSE in France than has been reported (Butler 1996). An appreciation of the possible underestimate of the number of cases of BSE in France can be made, paradoxically, by enquiring about the number of cows that died of something other than BSE. During the BSE epidemic in

Britain, all the cows that had clinical symptoms suggestive of BSE had to be killed and the brains examined to confirm the diagnosis. A proportion of cases that looked, clinically, as if they had BSE were found after death to have had another neurological disorder. The incidence of these other conditions can be expected to be fairly constant across time and between different countries which have similar farming practices. If the Europeans were examining every cow with the symptoms compatible with BSE, they would find these cases of 'BSE-like disease' even if they had no BSE at all in their country. As far as one can ascertain, the incidence of 'clinically suspect but neuropathologically negative cattle', that is, cattle with other neurological disease, in continental Europe, is very low. This suggests that the possibility of under-detection of BSE must be taken very seriously.

Another case of nvCJD with at least some florid plaques was subsequently reported from France, but, since the patient had been the recipient of a dura mater (meningeal) graft during previous neurosurgery, and since subsequent analysis of the prion protein revealed differences from nvCJD, it has to be supposed that this was an iatrogenic case rather than nvCJD. None the less, the confusion which this case has produced demonstrates that, while it may be possible to identify different types of CJD by describing the typical features of each type, individual cases often fall on the borderlines between these typical cases, and considerable clinical judgement has to be exercised in making a diagnosis. The claim that a monkey in a zoo in Montpelier had spontaneously developed spongiform encephalopathy, which might have suggested that zoo animal feed in continental Europe was contaminated, was subsequently challenged (Baker et al. 1996; Bons et al. 1996). In Britain, no monkeys fed on feedstuff containing the contaminated meat-and-bone meal associated with BSE have been reported to have developed prion disease. On a weight-for-weight basis the monkeys ate far more of the contaminated material than did the cows. The medical literature and the media are full of stories about 'prion diseases' in fox hounds in Britain, farmed ostriches in Germany, free-range lions in Africa, and parrots. If these cases are genuine, the implications for understanding the extent of the occurrence of prion disease are profound, but overwhelmingly convincing evidence of the nature of the disease in these cases is not available. Indeed, our colleague, Tony Palmer, examined the fox hounds and tells us that these animals did not have spongiform encephalopathy. Most of the cases in unusual animals are probably misdiagnoses, but they might not all be.

Was nvCJD really new?

Was it remotely possible that nvCJD was not a new disease but had always occurred at a rate of about one case per 10 million of the population? Clinical entities appear, and sometimes disappear, as the boundaries between one disease pattern and another move about. Until recently, an age at onset of less than 30 years would have been enough, in itself, to exclude the possibility that a disease was CJD. Unless prion disease is suspected, it could easily be misdiagnosed. Even the spongiform encephalopathy in the brain, which is regarded as highly characteristic of CJD, could be misinterpreted as the consequence of a metabolic disorder or certain other very rapidly progressive neurodegenerative diseases. PrP immunohistochemistry is a specialized technique used to prove a patient has had prion disease, once it has been suspected. Such techniques are not used routinely in cases in which a diagnosis of prion disease is not already being entertained. It is interesting that using the established diagnostic criteria, none of the nvCJD cases were classified as 'probable' or 'definite' cases of CJD prior to examination of brain material. Seven of the 10 cases did not even achieve a criterion of 'possible' CJD, one was classified as 'possible' CJD and the remaining two were identified first on the basis of examination of brain biopsy material. All these cases (except one, where permission for a post-mortem was not given by the next of kin) became 'definite' CJD only after the brain was examined. It is to the credit of the CJD Surveillance Unit that they managed to find something as important as nvCJD, even though it was not exactly what they were looking for.

There have been so few cases of nvCJD that any individual case is likely to have been the first that any doctor would have seen. When a patient presents with a pattern of symptoms that has never been seen before, most doctors would be reluctant to write it up as a new disease entity until there were other cases. Without the CJD Surveillance Unit, which was specifically set up to alert doctors to possible new presentations for CJD and to collate such cases, it is possible that nvCJD would have gone unreported. Interestingly, the announcement of the 10 cases of nvCJD did not result in doctors reporting similar cases that they had also seen recently, but had not known quite how to interpret. The CJD Surveillance Unit started collecting data in 1990 but the first cases of nvCJD were not found until 1994. The lack of cases of nvCJD between 1990 and 1994 found either at the time, by the CJD Surveillance Unit, or reported retrospectively by other neurologists, suggests that these new cases really did not exist before 1994.

How could nvCJD be related to BSE?

The British government had been issuing assurances for several years prior to 1996 that British beef was safe to eat. These assurances included Mr John Selwyn Gummer (the then Minister of Agriculture) attempting to prove his point by feeding his 6-year-old daughter, Cordelia, a hamburger in front of the television cameras. Unfortunately, the child appeared to burn her tongue on the meat and the publicity stunt was not well received. More prudent politicians were heard to say that the scientists had advised that the risk to human health was exceedingly small. Even this more cautious wording covered up two serious difficulties. The first was that these statements were usually made when some new piece of legislation such as the 'Specified Offals Ban' had just been put in place. Since the new legislation contained the measures that the scientific advice suggested were necessary, then, obviously, this was believed to be what was required to ensure that human health was protected. The politicians could then honestly say that they believed beef to be safe from that time on. Clearly they must have had some doubts about the conditions prevailing up to that time, otherwise they would not have inflicted another costly and difficult restriction on the beef industry. Few politicians, and even fewer scientists, were prepared to say that beef had always been safe.

The second difficulty seems to have been a fundamental misunderstanding that occurred between the scientific advisers and the politicians. The scientists, for the most part, advised that the risk of cross-species transmission of prion disease by the oral route, using material from an animal which was not yet overtly sick, was very low, and that, after the specified offals (especially the brain and spinal cord) had been removed from human food, the risk was 'remote'. Looked at from the viewpoint of a scientist trying to get an experiment to work, the chance of getting oral transmission across a species barrier, using muscle or non-specified offals from an apparently healthy animal, was indeed remote. By this they meant that perhaps only one out of several hundred or thousand recipient animals would get sick. In fact, it has never been demonstrated. However, the politicians needed to know what the risk was of *any of 50 million people* potentially exposed to contaminated food becoming ill. This is a completely different question. Since the announcement of the occurrence of ten cases of nvCJD in the preceding 2 years, the number of additional cases in the following year was another six. One in 10 million cases per year is a 'remote' risk to a scientist. Indeed, if BSE had caused a form of CJD which was indistinguishable from sporadic CJD, it would have gone undetected. Nevertheless, one in 10 million cases per year proved to be a wholly unacceptable consumer risk (even though this is rather less than the risk of being run over on the way to the butcher's shop to buy the meat) and was, therefore, politically unacceptable.

The British Government had accepted, in 1989, that the brain and spinal cord, together with certain other offals, were the tissues most likely to be contaminated with the agent of BSE in sick animals, and that eating such tissues could, in theory, be a risk to humans. Consequently, the Government concluded, in 1996 that the most likely source of contamination leading to nvCJD was from specified offals legally included in human food before 1989. Such offals should have come only from cattle with no visible signs of illness because all affected and suspect cattle had had to be destroyed since 1988. It has to be admitted, however, that the epidemiology of BSE suggests that cows became infected with BSE shortly after birth and were therefore incubating the disease for most of their life before they became sick at 4–5 years of age. Infectivity levels were believed to rise throughout the incubation period so that a cow incubating BSE, and slaughtered for food shortly before it became sick, would be expected to have carried considerable infectivity in its brain and spinal cord. Thus, some infectious, specified offals would have been eaten before 1989. Against this, it should be remembered that 'best beef' is eaten at less than 30 months old (when infectivity would be expected to be extremely low), and comes from beef herds where the incidence of BSE had always been much lower than in dairy herds. Dairy cows which are no longer economically useful could also be eaten, provided they had no signs of illness as a result of which they would have been judged unfit for human consumption. So material from dairy cows about to develop the symptoms of BSE, and therefore carrying high levels of infectious agent in the brain and spinal cord, would sometimes have been eaten by humans. Infectivity has only been found in brain and spinal cord of naturally infected cattle. No infectivity has been detected in muscle, which is what is usually meant by 'meat'.

Did people actually eat the brain and spinal cord? A little-known piece of legislation, the 'Meat and Spreadable Fish Products Regulations, 1984' banned the inclusion of a variety of meat offals, including brain and spinal cord, and other unappetizing meat and fish products in food sold raw. This legislation preceded the first case of BSE and was brought in for reasons unconnected with BSE. None the less, it had the effect of banning the use of bovine brain and spinal cord in mince, sausages, and hamburgers, sold raw or frozen, in supermarkets and butcher's shops. In practice, such products sold cooked would also have been protected by the same legislation if, at the time of manufacture, the state of the product on sale was not wholly prescribed. Major outlets of cooked hamburgers usually used products which were 100 per cent meat, that is, muscle, since this produced least shrinkage on cooking. The widespread belief that the most risky products were mince, sausages, and hamburgers was therefore unfounded.

Another source of concern was 'mechanically recovered meat'. In this process meat is stripped away from bone using jets of water and it was supposed that, if brain and spinal cord had not been adequately removed, it would be caught by this procedure and included as a bulking agent in cooked gravies, soups, meat pastes, etc. But brain tissue was unlikely to be included because the animal's head was not subject to this procedure (apparently the teeth would fall out and jam up the machine!). It was, however, possible that the membrane that surrounds the spinal cord and which adheres to the bones of the vertebral column could have been included in mechanically recovered meat. Such membranes are not known to be a risk, but they are similar to the meningeal membranes which surround the brain and which carry infectivity in affected humans.

How could it be proved that nvCJD was BSE-related?

There are three ways in which it may be possible to establish whether nvCJD is caused by BSE. The first involves creating transgenic mice which carry the human PrP gene and seeing whether they are susceptible to infection with BSE. This sort of experiment has already begun and the results so far have been somewhat surprising. It was found that BSE would transmit to transgenic mice which carried extra copies of the human PrP gene, in addition to the normal mouse PrP gene, with an incubation period that was similar to that found using normal mice (Collinge *et al.* 1995). But when the PrP^{sc} from these mice was analysed it was found to contain only mouse PrP not human PrP. In other words the transmission of BSE to mice had proceeded in such a way that the PrP molecules produced by the mouse PrP gene had become involved in the disease, whereas the much larger number of PrP molecules produced by the multiple copies of the human PrP gene had not been involved in the disease. Unfortunately, the human PrP gene, chosen for insertion in the mouse, had coded for valine at position 129, whereas all the nvCJD cases reported in the first instance were homozygous for methionine at position 129 of the PrP gene. Since there is now evidence to suggest that PrP molecules of different amino acid sequence compete with each other in complex ways, it will be necessary to run this sort of experiment again using transgenic mice that carry only the human PrP gene, and from which the mouse PrP gene has been removed. Very recently a report from Collinge's laboratory indicates that both BSE and nvCJD transmit to transgenic mice carrying copies of the human PrP gene (with valine at codon 129) but in which the mouse PrP gene has been removed. These mice showed similar behavioural signs (including walking backwards!), which differed from those shown by the same mice injected with brain material from other types of CJD patient (Hill *et al.* 1997).

The second way of assessing whether nvCJD is BSE-related is to carry out what are called 'strain typing' experiments. Transmission of prion disease to mice of different PrP genotypes produces a characteristic pattern of incubation periods in the different mice, and different distributions of neuropathology within the brains of different types of mouse. These data are used to define the strain of agent as it was in the donor animal. It so turns out that, whereas transmission from sheep scrapie results in the detection of many different strains of scrapie, transmissions from several different cows with BSE, collected from different geographical locations and at different times during the epidemic, all produced the same strain of agent. Even when BSE has passed through another species, such as the cats or exotic antelopes that have become sick as part of the BSE epidemic, the same strain of agent has been isolated from all these animals. This strain has not been found in any affected animal other than those associated with BSE. So, if the cases of nvCJD were caused by BSE, they too would be found to have the same strain of agent. Experiments to test this were set up shortly after the announcement about nvCJD, and the results have now been published (Bruce *et al.* 1997). New variant CJD produced a distribution of pathology in the mice which was indistinguishable from that produced in mice injected with BSE, and different from that produced in mice injected with material from sporadic cases of CJD.

The third way of assessing whether nvCJD is BSE-related is to do 'PrP-typing' experiments. One of the ways of demonstrating that a disease is a prion disease is to extract PrP^{sc} from brain tissue from the affected animal or person. Part of the procedure for doing this involves treating the brain tissue with the enzyme proteinase K, which digests most proteins, including PrP^{c}, away to nothing. PrP^{sc} is only partially sensitive to proteinase K and leaves a residue known as PrP27–30. The molecular weight of this fragment varies slightly according to the source. An analysis of molecular weight yields what has been described as a molecular 'signature' or PrP^{sc}-type. In the initial report of this analysis, sporadic or iatrogenic cases of CJD were all found to contain type 1, type 2, or type 3 PrP^{sc}. Cases that carried at least one valine at codon 129 were more likely to contain type 2 or type 3 PrP^{sc} than type 1 PrP^{sc}, which was found mainly in extracts from patients who were homozygous methionine at codon 129. All the new variant CJD cases produced type 4 PrP^{sc}, as did a cow with BSE, and a kudu, a monkey, and a cat, all with BSE-related disease, and mice experimentally infected with BSE (Collinge *et al.* 1996). The one case of nvCJD from France was subsequently also found to produce type 4 PrP^{sc}. These findings might look like conclusive proof that nvCJD is BSE-related, but there are a few problems. First, the types of PrP^{sc} extracted from different species still retain certain differences. For example, type 4 PrP^{sc} from cows with BSE will transmit with ease to mice and produce mouse type 4 PrP^{sc}; whereas type 4 PrP^{sc} from nvCJD has yet to transmit to mice. Secondly, PrP^{sc} type can change on transmission from one species to another, under conditions which are not fully defined, but which may depend on the PrP gene of the host. For example, type 1 PrP^{sc} from sporadic CJD cases, which were homozygous for methionine at codon 129, produced type 2 PrP^{sc} when transmitted to transgenic mice carrying multiple copies of the human PrP gene with valine at codon 129. Thirdly, while the results so far in humans are extremely interesting, it is necessary to look at PrP^{sc} types from as many backgrounds as possible.

At a press conference after the data were published, John Collinge said that the type 4 PrP^{sc} pattern was a molecular signature of BSE-related prion protein which provided additional evidence that the cases of new variant CJD were indeed BSE-related. With the new results of Bruce *et al.* (1997) and Hill *et al.* (1997), all but the most stubborn sceptics are now convinced that nvCJD is indeed BSE-related. We certainly are now convinced.

A second group of scientists (Parchi *et al.* 1997) has since published a comparable analysis of PrP^{sc} type. They confirmed that the PrP^{sc} type seen in one case of new variant CJD differed from that found in all their other cases, but they found only two types of PrP^{sc} in sporadic and iatrogenic cases of CJD and kuru. They did confirm that cases carrying at least one valine at codon 129 tended to produce different PrP^{sc} from cases that were homozygous for methionine at codon 129.

Can we assess how many more cases of nvCJD there will be?

The simple answer to this question is no. The BSE epidemic (in terms of observed cases) began in 1986 when six cows were affected. Subsequently a

Fragment weight kDa

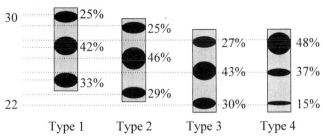

Fig. 9.3 This diagram attempts to explain PrP^{sc} typing and is based on the experiments of Collinge *et al.* (1996). Each column shows the result of digesting PrP^{sc} with proteinase K and separating the three major fragments (indicated by black blobs) according to the molecular weight of the fragment. This is done by allowing them to migrate through a gel in an electric field. (The lower the band in the diagram, the lighter the fragment). The lowest molecular weight band corresponds to the base fragment with no glycosyl side-chains, the middle band corresponds to the base fragment with one glycosyl side-chain, and the highest molecular weight band corresponds to the base fragment with two glycosyl side-chains. Types 1, 2, and 3 differ in the molecular weights of the base fragments but not in the percentages of the three glycoforms. Type 4 differs from type 3 in that although the base fragment molecular weight is the same as for type 3, the percentages of the glycoforms differ. The PrP^{sc} extracted from sporadic CJD is usually type 1 or type 2, and that from a few cases of ghCJD has been found to be usually type 3. Type 4 PrP^{sc} has been found in cattle with BSE, animals to which BSE has been transmitted, either experimentally or by feed contamination, and in humans with new variant CJD.

few cows that had died before 1986 were investigated, and it seems very likely that a handful of cases occurred in 1985 and perhaps 1984. From 1986 to 1987 the number of affected cows increased almost tenfold and rose substantially in 1988 and again in 1989. If nvCJD was BSE-related, the number of cases diagnosed would be expected to follow a similar pattern a number of years later. However, the rate of increase would probably be much lower because an additional variation in incubation period would be added to the curve of increasing exposure. This pattern is not affected by whether the risk comprises eating tissue from affected or merely incubating cattle, or whether the risk came from just brain, or other tissues as well, because all the events of the epidemic are linked to the pattern of occurrence of cases of BSE. If BSE transmits readily to people with an incubation period of more than 10 years, the 10 cases of nvCJD in 1994–95 could be the consequence of eating contaminated material from a very few cows affected before 1985. If this is the case, the implications for the occurrence of an epidemic of nvCJD occurring more than 10 years after the period between 1986 (when only a handful of BSE cases occurred) and the imposition of the Specified Offals Ban in November 1989 (when about 7000 cases of BSE occurred in the preceding 12 months) are horrendous.

It could equally well be the case, however, that BSE transmits to humans only with the greatest difficulty, and that the nvCJD cases represent the very few individuals who were sufficiently sensitive to infection (for some reason), or who were so exceptionally exposed that they acquired the disease at the height of the BSE epidemic before the Specified Offals Ban. This would have been during most of 1989. The incubation period would then be about 5–6 years. Since the risk of exposure would have been greatly reduced by the Specified Offals Ban, it could be argued that there will not be very more cases.

When the first 10 cases of nvCJD were announced in March 1996, many people, ourselves included, suggested that if nvCJD was BSE-related, a rise in the number of cases would appear in the subsequent 12 months. By March 1997 a few people were beginning to ask 'what epidemic?'. While the fact that there were only six more cases in the following year is reassuring, it does not imply that there will not be a large epidemic. Because the potential incubation period is unknown, it may be several years before the magnitude of any epidemic can be realistically assessed. Anything else is guesswork.

Who is at risk?

The first 10 cases of nvCJD were all homozygous for methionine at codon 129 of the PrP gene. If subsequent cases of nvCJD are the same, a substantial proportion of the population may be protected against nvCJD, since only 37 per cent of the White European population is homozygous for methionine at codon 129 of the PrP gene. It is possible, however, that as time goes by nvCJD will begin to occur in people who are homozygous for valine at codon 129 and will eventually occur in people who are heterozygous. By analogy with iatrogenic and sporadic CJD, it would seem likely that heterozygotes will be somewhat protected against nvCJD. This is, however, no consolation since a disease that affected half the population would be catastrophic. If the incubation period is in excess of 10 years, the very elderly will not be affected, because they will die of old age first, but this is scarcely any consolation.

We may suppose that the first people to develop illness would be those who were exposed to an exceptionally large amount of infectivity. To our knowledge, little attempt has been made to establish how evenly infectivity could have been spread through human food. It is here that the assumption that mince, sausages, and hamburgers are the major culprit becomes dangerous. As we said earlier, the Meat and Spreadable Fish Products Regulations, 1984, should have prevented the inclusion of brain tissue in these products. Let us suppose, however, that 'lumps' of brain from affected or incubating cows were included in some meat products. Such 'lumps' would be spread very unevenly through human food so that it would be a matter of extreme bad luck for those who ate these isolated 'packets of infectivity'. It is possible, however, that infectivity is spread much more evenly and thinly throughout human food. Many products, including sweets, puddings, and other products, not usually thought of as containing 'meat', nevertheless contain beef-derived ingredients. The amount of beef-derived material in such products is likely to be extremely small, but if the infectious agent has been separated out in such a way as to find its way into these products, it may be supposed that a large proportion of the population has been exposed to an extremely low level of infectivity. 'A very low level of infectivity' means that only a very small proportion of people exposed to that level of infectivity will get sick, although it will not be possible to predict who they will be. Apart from being young, the first 10 cases of nvCJD did not share any special features of diet or habit which would lead one to predict which type of people are at risk.

Since the BSE epidemic will have lasted for about 15 years in Britain, it is to be predicted that any epidemic of CJD which is caused by BSE will last for the same length of time plus the variation in incubation time which results in humans from variable levels of exposure. In kuru, the incubation period probably ranged from 3 to 30 years, with the very last handful of cases having an incubation period in excess of 40 years. In theory, anyone consuming the infectious agent during the BSE epidemic is likely to be at risk for a substantial proportion of the rest of their life. If a BSE epidemic of any great magnitude were to occur in other European countries, and it is our view that this is quite likely, the risk to humans will extend well into the next century. Against all this gloom one should, none the less, remember that although the link between nvCJD and BSE is now accepted, the extent of the exposure of humans is not known and may be small. As time passes it will become clear from the epidemiological pattern of occurrence of cases what the future holds. The pattern of occurrence of prion disease is frequently surprising but, like the pattern of occurrence of AIDS, it never lies.

So what went wrong?

The beef industry in Britain has been ruined, the rendering industry is in chaos, the dairy industry is in deep trouble, and the presumption is that people have died as a result of eating contaminated food. Many more people may die in the future. Undeniably BSE has been a disaster and, with the benefit of hindsight, it is easy to see that things could have been done differently. The media has promulgated the view that all aspects of the BSE epidemic have been caused by incompetence, negligence, or malevolent self-interest. Although human beings are never perfect and mistakes have been made, the fiendish nature of the infectious agent of prion disease and the logistical difficulties of making the right decisions in a situation where it takes 5 years to find out whether what you did was appropriate present enormous difficulties.

Could the BSE epidemic have been avoided?

There are many areas where it may now be impossible to establish what actually happened. One example of this is the *origin* of BSE. Scientific experiments can be performed to establish the plausibility of certain events, for example, whether sheep scrapie, transmitted orally to cows produces a disease that is identical to BSE. If it does not, this brings into question whether scrapie was the source of BSE in Britain, but it cannot prove what happened as a historical event. The major change that occurred in the rendering industry in the early 1980s (when the first cows destined to get BSE were born) was from batch processing to continuous processing. This new method did not involve the use of solvent extraction to remove the last remaining fat content and was run at a lower temperature. The continuous processing method had been used in other countries without ill effect, the temperatures involved in the new system were more than adequate to inactivate all known bacteria and viruses, and the specific protective effect afforded by the remaining fat was not known. But the inability of the new system to inactivate the infectious agent of scrapie and BSE could not be predicted, and the switch to the new system, while economically advantageous, was not undertaken as a direct consequence of 'deregulation' or as a result of negligence. That Britain had a very high level of scrapie was unfortunate but scrapie was, and still is, regarded as being non-hazardous to humans, and the massive economic cost of attempting to eradicate scrapie at that time far outweighed the economic cost of scrapie to the sheep-based industries. Plans to eradicate scrapie have now been instigated because it might be impossible to distinguish between natural scrapie and a spongiform encephalopathy in sheep infected with the 'BSE' agent. Such a disease might retain its infectivity to other animals including, possibly, man. The eradication of scrapie has also been made feasible by the development of molecular genetic techniques which now make it possible to identify sheep that are highly susceptible to natural scrapie.

Could the BSE epidemic have been brought to an end more quickly?

This question can be broken down into several components. Were the right policies put in place to eradicate BSE? Were they adequately enforced, monitored, and complied with? Was there incompetence, negligence, or malpractice? Could it all have been done more quickly? The answer to the latter is almost certainly yes although, even if everything had been done at breakneck speed, it might not have made a great deal of difference. This is because the 5-year incubation period of BSE means that there was a delay of 5 years during which the BSE epidemic was becoming silently established in up to 200 000 cattle before anything was visible. (The majority of these infected cattle would never show symptoms because they would be killed before reaching the age of onset.) The inadequacy of any legislative measure designed to curb BSE would not become apparent for 5 years after it was put in place. In these circumstances, speeding up the legislative measures by a few months would have helped, but it would not have stopped the epidemic in its tracks. Until March 1996, all legislation was based on the need to eradicate BSE because the loss of confidence in beef by the British public was causing economic losses to the cattle industries and because BSE was a *theoretical* risk to humans (rather than a *known* risk). In the first case it would have been inappropriate for the legislation to be more expensive than the economic cost of the disease. In the second case a genuine ambivalence pervaded much discussion and decision making for many years. This ambivalence may account for the 16-month gap between the Ruminant Feed Ban in July 1988, which was designed to prevent cattle from being infected, and the Specified Bovine Offals Ban in November 1989, which was designed to prevent people from being infected. It would be absurd to argue that this meant that the Government cared more about cattle than people, although it does indicate that they did not believe at that time that BSE was a risk to humans. At the same time as the Ruminant Feed Ban came into force, the inclusion of any part of the carcass of a cow with (or suspected of having) BSE in human food had been banned. The Specified Bovine Offals Ban applied to all adult cattle and was designed to protect the public from the possible risk of infection from healthy cattle incubating BSE. Even now doubt remains that new variant CJD is caused by eating contaminated food. After March 1996 most of the legislative changes, including the '30 Month Scheme', were designed to restore confidence in British beef rather than to protect the public health. Again, this was not because no-one cared about the public health but rather was because the Specified Bovine Offals Ban of 1989, and subsequent tightening of that legislation, had already covered everything that reasonably could be done to protect health on the basis of all the scientific evidence. The view in March 1996 was that the most likely explanation for the occurrence of the new variant of CJD was that 'these cases are linked to BSE *before the introduction of the Specified Bovine Offals Ban of 1989'*. This remains the supposition.

Were the right policies put in place to eradicate BSE?

In the period from the imposition of the Ruminant Feed Ban (1988) to the Specified Bovine Offals Ban (1989) the number of cows born which subsequently developed BSE fell by more than 90 per cent from the predicted number that would have been born if the Ruminant Feed Ban had not been put in place. This was quite an achievement, although, clearly, it was not enough. Failures to implement the legislation must have occurred, and these can be laid at the feet of those whose job it was to do this and those whose job it was to monitor and enforce this legislation. The policy of removing ruminant-derived material from ruminant feedstuff produced a decrease in the birth of new cases of BSE to negligible levels by 1992, even though this was against a background of a sharply rising number of new cases becoming sick. This suggests that there was a considerable amount of contaminated material 'in the pipeline', that is, stored in half-processed form as ingredients ready for incorporation in different feedstuffs by compounders, or in sacks of rendered material all over the country ready for distribution, and so on. More than a million tons of material is rendered every year, and while it might have been possible to 'recall' some of it, it would have been impossible to destroy all potentially infected material overnight. The disposal of such large quantities of material would have produced major difficulties. Burning it might have led to the production of illegal levels of smoke and carbon dioxide. Animal husbandry is so dependent on pelleted feedstuffs that it is not clear what commercial animals would have been fed on if rendered material had been banned overnight. The Specified Bovine Offals Ban, though designed primarily to protect human health, may have had the added advantage of ensuring that more of the specified bovine offals were actually destroyed rather than being used for other purposes, where cross-contamination might have occurred. There was evidence that specified bovine offals, legally processed for inclusion in pig and poultry feed, was finding its way through cross-contamination back into feedstuff for cows. This was detected by John Wilesmith working at the Central Veterinary Laboratory as a geographical association between cases of BSE born after the Ruminant Feed Ban and the number of pigs and poultry in different parts of the country. Subsequent legislation was then able to remove this potential source of contamination.

Were the policies to eradicate BSE adequately enforced, monitored, and complied with or was there incompetence, negligence, and malpractice?

More than 33 000 cattle born after the Ruminant Feed Ban have developed BSE. These are described as BABs (born-after-the-ban). Since the Ruminant Feed Ban was intended to prevent the occurrence of these BABs something clearly went wrong. As we have already suggested, the steady decline in the proportion of cows born between the time of the Ruminant Feed Ban and the Specified Offals Ban which subsequently went on to get BSE is not due to a decrease in the amount of infected material which might otherwise have been fed to cattle, because the number of cases of BSE being diagnosed was increasing during that period. Rather this decline suggests that the monitoring and enforcement of the Ruminant Feed Ban got off to an inadequate start but improved throughout that time. Compliance probably also improved as people began to realize that the legislation had 'bite' and that the whole situation was very serious. In June 1997, following a survey of compliance with regulations designed to combat BSE throughout Europe, Franz Fischler, the European Commissioner for Agriculture, said that Great Britain was the only member of the European Community that appeared to be complying with these regulations. Nevertheless, within a week of Fischler's remarks being made, evidence was emerging about the illegal export of British beef to continental Europe.

Could research have been done more quickly?

Research is expensive and much of the money used for research comes from the taxpayer. Research proposals are very carefully scrutinized. In some funding schemes, particularly those used by the universities, a scientist decides what he or she want to do and applies for the money to do it. In other funding schemes, especially those operating in institutions directly funded by government departments, research areas are identified and scientists are asked to solve particular problems. In both systems, decision making about research proposals and the allocation of money can take up to a year. Such systems as these have difficulty providing scientific answers in a political time frame. Research on animals is particularly bureaucratic. For example, the apparently simple business of collecting blood samples from a large number of normal cows is problematic because such work requires a Home Office licence for experimentation on animals and experiments have to be done on designated animals in designated laboratories. Such problems are not insurmountable but they do slow down the planning necessary to undertake large experiments. Funding systems which respond to scientists' ideas run the risk of generating research which the general public regards as irrelevant and occasionally frivolous. Funding systems which identify problems to be solved do not invariably produce scientific advance. The Ministry of Agriculture, Food and Fisheries (MAFF) spent hundreds of thousands of pounds searching for a simple test (for example, a blood test) which would make it possible to identify cows that were going to develop BSE but which, at the time, were not producing infectious agent. Even better, they would have liked a test that would tell them which cows were definitely not infected and were therefore safe to eat or to export to Europe. No such test has become available during the course of the BSE epidemic. This is not because of a lack of effort, but because being infected, producing infectious agent, and manifesting physiological or biochemical indicators of infection are intimately linked.

Was there secrecy?

The media are very fond of claiming that there was a 'cover-up' about BSE. There was undoubtedly a desire not to cause economically damaging alarm at a time when it was not clear that there was anything to be alarmed about. This may occasionally have spilt over into a desire to keep facts out of the public domain for fear of the political consequences, but it is clear that much of what the media complained about was justifiable confidentiality. Bob Will at the CJD Surveillance Unit tells us that he has never been under any pressure from any government body to withhold data about CJD, and particularly the new variant of CJD. But he has been under pressure from journalists to reveal the names and addresses of people with CJD and of people for whom the diagnosis was still under consideration. Such personal, medical information is absolutely confidential, and no medical practitioner would reveal such information since it would not be in the patient's interest to do so.

When we succeeded in transmitting first scrapie and then BSE to monkeys, we conveyed our findings immediately to the Tyrrell Committee (the forerunner of SEAC) on 27 February 1992. A decision was taken to put the result in 'the public domain' as quickly as possible. This was done on 5 March 1992 by way of a statement to the House of Commons about the experimental host range of BSE. The scientific publication of this work appeared in *Veterinary Record* on 17 April 1993. The delay between these two events was mainly because of the lengthy process by which manuscripts are reviewed by other scientists and revisions are suggested. We were approached by several journalists during that delay who were convinced that we had been prevented from publishing the work because of some sort of censorship. This was not the case.

Science is about the interpretation of data and many scientists are reluctant to publish until they have had time to think about the right interpretation. They will often want to run other experiments which will make interpretation more sound. While the media were complaining of lack of publication, many scientists working on BSE felt that they were under too much pressure to publish or share their data before they were ready. This was so in the case of the 7-year bovine maternal transmission experiment run by the Central Veterinary Laboratory and described earlier. The experiment was run 'blind', that is, with the cows identified only by numbers, so that no one looking after them or examining their brains after death, knew whether or not they been born of a mother who later developed BSE. It should have been concluded in late 1996 when the youngest cows had reached 7 years of age. But during the summer of 1996 there was so much concern that BSE might be passed from cow to calf that, with great reluctance, the scientists 'broke the code' and examined how many of the cows with BSE had mothers which also died of BSE. These data were then submitted to *Nature* for publication. The data were also made available to epidemiologists in Oxford who submitted another paper to *Nature* in which they presented calculations of the efficiencies of various slaughter policies, based in part *on the assumption that maternal transmission of BSE was one of the factors that contributed to the persistence of BSE in the cattle population* (Anderson *et al.* 1996). Unfortunately, further consideration of the results of the maternal transmission experiment led some investigators, ourselves included, to suggest that the experiment could not distinguish between maternal transmission of the infectious agent itself and inheritance of genetic susceptibility to disease. The authors of the first paper decided not to publish, to allow time for yet further analysis. However, the paper by Anderson and his colleagues was published and refers to the withdrawn paper as being *submitted* when in fact it does not exist. This unfortunate state of affairs would not have occurred if the scientists who carried out the original experiment had not been put under unreasonable pressure to publish or to distribute their hard-earned data. They certainly cannot be accused of secrecy.

Funding systems that allow scientists to pursue their own ideas generate a very competitive atmosphere. Researchers are keen to publish as frequently as possible, since this enables them to be seen as productive and therefore deserving of funds. A disadvantage of these systems is that they favour short-term, small-scale projects in which as many publications as possible are generated from as little work as possible. The advantage is that data are fully presented in the scientific journals and are therefore available to scientists, journalists, and others who have access to a scientific library. The funding system operating in some directly funded institutions and in parts of the scientific civil service allows important work to be done in areas which are of great value to human or animal health (as well as in other areas such as road safety or military defence) but which may be long term and may be more concerned with collecting valuable data (for example, monitoring disease incidence) than in exploring scientific hypotheses. This second method of funding is very important but it may not lead to rapid publication. Some of the research on BSE falls into this category and publication of some of the results has been frustratingly obscure. This may not be deliberate secrecy; rather it may represent the effect that a particular style of research management has on the final product.

Were the policies appropriate for the protection of human health?

After August 1988 any cow suspected of suffering from BSE had to be killed and the use of any part of the carcass in food for humans or animals was forbidden. In December 1988 the use of milk from any cow suspected of having BSE was also banned in food. Both of these actions resulted from interim advice given by the Southwood Committee before that committee made its full report to Ministers in February 1989. There was, at that time, no scientific evidence that BSE posed any greater risk to man than did scrapie, which was believed not to be hazardous to man. None the less, based on the possibility that BSE might be different from scrapie, it was decided to recommend that greater precautions be taken with BSE than with scrapie. At that time the risk of infection from apparently healthy cattle had not been fully addressed. The Southwood Committee appears not to have appreciated the ratio of infected but apparently healthy cattle to overtly sick animals, since on the basis of the number of known cases of BSE it suggested that the total epidemic would be of the order of 20 000 animals. In fact, the total number of cows diagnosed as having BSE in Britain will be nearer 180 000 by the end of the epidemic. Some of this difference results from the initial inefficiency of the Ruminant Feed Ban, but most of the cows destined to get BSE had already acquired the infection by the time the Southwood Committee made its report.

The amount of infectious agent in the various edible tissues of cows at different stages of the incubation period is obviously an important consideration in determining a policy to protect human health, if that infectivity can actually cross the species barrier to humans. This vital piece of information was very difficult to acquire. Experiments were set up to measure the distribution of infectivity in different tissues in affected cows, but such experiments take years to complete because they involve transmissions to other animals. They established that certain tissues, for example, brain and spinal cord, contain large amounts of infectivity by the time the cow is overtly sick, but this came as no surprise to anyone. What these experiments cannot do is provide assurance that other tissues, and tissues taken from cows early in the incubation period, are free of infectivity. While it is only necessary to get one successful transmission to show that infectivity is present, low levels of infectivity result in very low transmission rates so that an enormous number of transmission experiments would be needed to show that infectivity is probably not present. Even then, one could not be sure. Public-health decisions and scientific data were necessarily somewhat dissociated at the time legislation was put in place, but this was because of the political imperative to take urgent action against an unknown risk to humans rather than because of a disregard for scientific data.

Sadly, only time will tell whether the best measures to protect human health were taken. It must be recognized that legislation was not always put in place with as much speed as was possible; that the legislation did not always take into account the practicalities of enforcement, monitoring, and compliance; and that negligence and illegal acts must have occurred. But it would be foolish to argue that if all parties had behaved properly and the regulations had been fully implemented, it would have been possible to bring the epidemic to an immediate conclusion. The failure to find cases of new variant CJD dating from before the onset of the BSE epidemic, or in parts of the world not affected by BSE, was the only direct evidence that nvCJD is BSE-related. Laboratory evidence has now accumulated that nvCJD is indeed BSE-related. The number of cases of nvCJD in the next 40 or more years will tell us how big the risk has been. The number of cases occurring in people born after the imposition of the Specified Bovine Offals Ban will tell us how effective that measure was but, if nvCJD *is* BSE-related, then most of the investigators working on the BSE epidemic will not live long enough to see the end of the story.

10

What kind of disease is this?

We started this book by suggesting that prion disease was something new to biology. As a disease, of course, it has been with us for as long as we can know about and has presumably existed for thousands of years. We have had to move beyond conventional views of both virology and genetics in order to explain how a disease can be sometimes inherited or spontaneous, and sometimes acquired. We have argued that prion disease is unique and exciting, but part of the excitement lies in the possibility that prion disease will turn out *not* to be unique. An understanding of prion disease might provide insights into other biological processes and diseases.

Are prions alive?

What constitutes a living organism? Most animals, plants, fungi, and bacteria are capable of living and reproducing independently of other species, but parasitic organisms are dependent on other living organisms for their sustenance. In what way is the mistletoe, which draws nutrients from the tree in which it lodges, independent of that tree? The answer is that the mistletoe has a genome that is independent of the genome of the tree. The two genomes will compete with each other, since the mistletoe will evolve methods of extracting nutrients from the tree more efficiently, while the tree will develop methods of protecting itself from the demands of the mistletoe. Viruses are like parasites in that they cannot reproduce outside living cells and can usually only survive for short periods without the protection of a cellular system. They are considered to be independent of the host they infect because they contain nucleic acid and, therefore, *direct* their own replication, but they need the machinery of living cells in order to *make* copies of themselves. Although viruses are genetically independent of the hosts they infect, their evolutionary origin is obscure. Since the genetic code (the alphabetic relationship between codons and amino acids) is shared by viruses and larger organisms, it seems likely that viruses are made of bits of genetic material that 'escaped' from other living organisms and became independent.

Retroviruses (such as HIV) span the boundary between organisms and non-organisms. They behave like conventional viruses in that they can be transmitted from one organism to another, usually by the transfer of bodily fluids. They also contain some genetic material, which defines them as independent. Once a retrovirus enters a new cell, the genetic material contained in the retrovirus (in the form of RNA) uses a retrovirus-specific enzyme, called reverse transcriptase, to direct the synthesis of DNA, which is then inserted into the DNA of the infected cell. The inserted DNA, which is now part of the host, directs the manufacture of more retroviral particles, which ultimately kill the host.

There are bits of DNA, known as transposons, which exist within the genome, but which replicate themselves, so that multiple copies exist. These bits of DNA can be considered to be parasitic on the cellular DNA. When the cell divides, the transposons are reproduced in the genome of the daughter cells. They are therefore part of the genome of the cell, but since they can also replicate themselves, they can be considered to be at least partly independent of the cell. These anomalies blur the distinction between one organism and another. Similarly, prions are part of the host, since the PrP, of which they are made, is manufactured by the host, but their ability to cause infection in other animals, and the information held within them which determines strain characteristics, cannot be considered as belonging to the host, even though that information is not stored in the form of nucleic acid. Until recently, replication in biology and the information contained in DNA were thought to be totally interdependent. This is no longer thought to be the case by some biologists.

Richard Dawkins has pointed out that it is genes rather than organisms that replicate (Dawkins 1976). When two people produce a baby, that baby is genetically only 50 per cent like the father and 50 per cent like the mother. The baby is genetically unique, so neither the mother nor the father has, strictly speaking, reproduced. Half of the genes of each the parent, will however, be reproduced in the baby, albeit in a unique combination. Until recently, only identical twins had identical genomes, but the announcement in March 1997 that a sheep called Dolly had been 'cloned' at the Roslin Institute in Scotland changed all that. Dolly was made from the genetic material from one cell of another adult sheep and so was genetically identical to that other sheep. The reason why this has caused some consternation is that, in theory, it is now possible to clone human beings, so that, for example, a 'replacement' might be made for a dying child, or a man might decide that he would like his 'son and heir' to be identical to himself. This could place an intolerable psychological burden on the 'cloned' person. Using cloning techniques, it would be possible to produce hundreds of identical animals. This could be valuable if the animal had some special feature, but, equally, much damage could be done if that animal also turned out to have some bad traits. Because each gene is passed to half of any animal's offspring, genes can spread through a population like an infection in just a few generations. The whole species could be weakened if the usual genetic diversity, which exists within one species, was diminished by too much cloning.

To return to Richard Dawkins. He argues that what mattered in evolution, and, therefore, what defines independent life, is not the whole animal (the gene vehicle) or the genomic DNA itself, but the *information* carried by that DNA. Although DNA is used as a template from which new DNA molecules are made, it is actually the information that those molecules hold, rather than the molecules themselves, which is reproduced. Furthermore, information may be stored and reproduced by mechanisms other than those requiring DNA, and when this occurs, the information will 'behave' much like a living organism. The easiest example cited by Dawkins is the 'computer virus'. This is, of course, man-made, but consists of information within a computer program which instructs the program to do unpleasant things to the rest of the software, and sometimes hardware, of the computer, and to make copies of those instructions which will then move about in the rest of the software of the computer. These computer viruses 'infect', and sometimes disable, computers. If the programs in which they are concealed are transferred to another computer, the new computer will also be infected and will suffer the same fate. Computer programmers have since built 'immune systems' into computers, which can detect and inactivate the computer viruses. However, the people who invented the computer viruses (who must have particularly unpleasant personalities to want to cause damage and misery that they will never know about) have invented viruses that can 'mutate' and so escape the efforts of the computer 'immune systems' to destroy them.

Another form of replicating information that Dawkins describes is the 'meme'. The ideas behind this are complex, but the meme consists, essentially, of the changes that occur in the brain when a piece of information or an 'idea' is transferred from one brain to another. Although the neuronal changes that occur when we pick up an idea are not fully understood, it is likely that those neuronal changes that underlie an idea in one brain will be reproduced in another brain when people communicate. These neuronal changes are the memes, and they can replicate like infections. They also 'mutate' in that errors of understanding and reproduction occur. This can be seen in the game of 'Chinese whispers' in which half-heard messages undergo particularly rapid changes.

DNA, computer viruses, and 'memes' are very different storage systems. But once we accept that replicable information can be stored in different ways, we can explore the possibility that the information stored and replicated in prions can exist in something other than DNA. At least two other forms of biological information storage and replication that are independent of DNA have been identified in yeast. Two yeast proteins can take on different molecular shapes, the shape achieved depending on the shape of the protein molecules already present. There is even a suggestion that at least one of the proteins can take on multiple conformations (Derkatch et al. 1996). We could regard this as being equivalent to strains of agent in prion disease.

The existence of parasitic life forms shows that the distinction between one independent organism and another can be complex. The best way of defining independence in biology is by regarding bits of replicating information as independent 'units of life'. In most cases these are genes. Evolution occurs because genes compete with each other, so that some genes increase in number while others become extinct. This means that evolution and genetics are intimately linked, but it is worth considering the extent to which other sources of replicating information interact with genes and can also be considered to be 'units of life'. We will discuss the way in which genes interact to produce competition between organisms (which are made by collections of genes), and the way in which genes (particularly different copies of the prion gene) compete with prions. The point of doing this is to try to set prion disease in a wider biological context.

Why do we all die?

Sir Peter Medawar won the Nobel prize for medicine in 1960 for his work in the field of immunology. In his book *The uniqueness of the individual*, he provided an elegant explanation of why all organisms grow old and die (Medawar 1957). The lifespan of most organisms is curtailed by events that have nothing to do with age, for example accidents, infections, or predations. With the passage of time after birth, the more likely it is that an organism will already have succumbed to one of these events. Therefore, a gene that has a beneficial effect for the organism (animal or person) shortly after birth, is 'worth' more than one that promises a beneficial effect a long time after birth, because the animal or person may already have died before this beneficial effect is realized. Equally, a gene that has a deleterious effect early in life is more damaging than one that has deleterious effects later in life, so that a gene deleterious very late in life can hardly be regarded as harmful. Evolution would have difficulty eliminating a gene that invariably caused a fatal disease but which did not do so until a person was more than 100 years old. Over the course of evolution, genes that have beneficial effects early in life are strongly selected, while those whose beneficial effects occur only late in life are weakly selected. Genes that are fatal very early in life are eliminated (except as recessive genes), whereas genes that are deleterious late in life cannot be eliminated. Senescence consists of the accumulated effects of many deleterious genes that act late in life. We therefore develop the diseases of old age. These include particularly the consequences of the loss of those biological mechanisms that keep genes themselves in good order. One of the consequences of this is that the genetic control of cell division is lost and we develop cancers.

Why is the PrP gene the way it is?

Presumably, the PrP gene exists because normal prion protein is valuable to the host, although we do not know what function it fulfils. The gene is highly conserved across many species, implying that its function is probably very important and basic. In humans, the normal 'wild-type' PrP gene has a probability of producing prion disease of only one in a million people per year. This is extremely low and shows that natural selection has succeeded in producing a gene whose frailty in this respect has been reduced to a minimum. Spontaneous disease in association with the 'wild-type' PrP gene has not been reported in wild animals (except perhaps in mule deer) because they do not live long enough to exhibit such a disease of old age. Even in captivity, animals do not live long enough to develop prion disease. Commercial animals are not kept beyond the prime of life and most pet owners have the good sense to have their pets humanely killed when they become too old to be healthy.

There are, as we have seen, many mutations in the human PrP gene which lead to prion disease later in life. These mutations are, therefore, examples of what are known as 'senescence genes', that is, genes (strictly speaking, alleles) which persist in the population despite being lethal to the host because the lethal effect is only manifest after the host has had enough time to have had children. None the less, possession of a lethal PrP gene mutation is disadvantageous since it can cause disease before the end of reproductive capability. It may also jeopardize the survival of offspring in humans, since parental and even grandparental support is important in determining success in human evolution. It can be predicted from this that even as a senescence gene, mutations leading to prion disease will be rare, and this is the case. All the dominant mutations considered together cause disease at a rate of one in 10 million of the Western population and the rate is likely to be much lower in less prosperous countries (and in former times), when longevity was curtailed by many other diseases and disasters.

All the genes of one organism are bound together in the sense that a gene that kills its host kills all the other genes in that host as well. Genes will therefore be in competition with each other to protect themselves from the disadvantageous effects of one of their number. Thus the genome contains 'gene modifiers', that is, genes that dilute out the effects of 'bad' genes, either by reducing their effects or by delaying the onset of the bad effects of those genes until old age. In the case of dominant genes (where one mutant copy of the gene is enough to cause bad effects), gene modifiers are most effective in delaying the onset of those bad effects, that is, in turning those 'bad' genes into 'senescence' genes. Humans possess a large number of senescence genes which cause late-onset disorders such as Alzheimer's disease and Huntington's disease. The mutations that cause prion disease belong with these other late-onset, dominantly inherited disorders.

Recessive genes, that is, those that cause disease only when there are two identical mutant copies, escape the effects of selective pressure in that they have no deleterious effect whenever they occur as only one copy in a genome. The mutant copy of the gene responsible for cystic fibrosis can pass silently from one person to another for many generations without noticeable effect. Only when two people who both carry a mutant copy of that gene marry and produce a child, who carries two mutant copies, will disease occur. In this case, however, selective pressure has had little chance to increase the age of onset of the bad effects of that mutant copy because there is no selective pressure acting in those people who only carry one mutant copy of the gene. Recessive disorders, like cystic fibrosis, therefore tend to have an onset in childhood. Rather ironically, 'mature' recessive disorders, that is, those that began thousands of years ago and on which selective pressure has had the most effect, will have a very early onset because the very early death of a child increases the chances of the parents having more children, some of whom will carry one mutant copy of the gene and will therefore perpetuate the survival of that mutation. Scrapie in sheep seems to behave as an 'immature' recessive disorder. Sheep carrying two copies of a scrapie-related mutation in the PrP gene develop scrapie in early adulthood, whereas a very few sheep with only one copy of that mutation will develop scrapie in old age.

Some genes can be described as 'Faustian genes' in that they are specifically beneficial in early life but lethal later. Scrapie-associated mutations in sheep may fall into this category. Scrapie became common in the eighteenth century because sheep breeders selected sheep on the basis of good traits in lambs (weight gain, sturdiness, and so on) only to find that they had inadvertently chosen sheep that developed scrapie later in life.

Gene modifiers are also important in scrapie. The recessive mutation in the PrP gene which leads to scrapie in Suffolk sheep is not associated with scrapie in Cheviot sheep, suggesting that there is something about the Cheviot genome (which may lie somewhere else in the PrP gene or in another gene) which protects the Cheviot sheep from the effects of this mutation.

We said at the beginning of this section that the PrP gene was conserved because it had value to the host unconnected with its involvement in prion disease. This must explain how the gene evolved in the first place, but there is another peculiar way in which the PrP gene might be conserved. Dominant mutations in the PrP gene which led to prion disease in childhood or in the fetus could not be inherited, because carriers of this gene would have no children of their own. Such mutations will, therefore, not be found in the population. This will limit the amount of variation in the gene and contribute to its conservation in ways which have nothing to do with the value of the gene to the host. In this respect, the PrP gene could be described as a 'blackmail' gene .

Although different copies of the same gene compete with each other, they occasionally support each other. This rather unusual phenomenon is known as 'heterozygote advantage'. The best-known example of this is a mutation in the gene that makes one of the components of the chemical haemoglobin, which carries oxygen around in the blood. This mutation causes a disease called sickle-cell anaemia, which is common in people who come from those parts of Africa that have, or used to have, very high levels of malaria. Sickle-cell anaemia is a recessive disorder which is frequently fatal. But why is it common in malaria-infested parts of Africa? It has been found that people who carry just one mutant copy of the haemoglobin gene are partially resistant to malaria, which can also be fatal if not treated, so that they have a genetic advantage over people who carry two normal copies of the haemoglobin gene. Heterozygotes who carry one copy of the normal gene and one mutant copy do not die of either malaria or sickle-cell anaemia and are, therefore, described as having heterozygote advantage. In humans, sporadic or acquired prion disease is much less common in people who are heterozygous for the polymorphism at codon 129 of the PrP gene than in people who are homozygous for either methionine or valine at codon 129. The occurrence of both methionine and valine at codon 129 may, therefore, be maintained in the population by the mechanism of heterozygote advantage.

Prion disease fights back

We have described various ways in which the prion gene, though a prerequisite for the development of prion disease, has been subjected to various evolutionary pressures to ensure that prion disease is rare, recessive, or restricted to old age. If infectious prion proteins contain replicable information, they can be expected to fight back in order to survive, and the most conspicuous way in which this occurs is through their transmissibility. Prion disease occurs in two epidemiological patterns, endemic and epidemic disease. Diseases are described as endemic when they occur at a constant level throughout a population. In the case of prion disease this occurs only in humans and sheep, where the *endemic* occurrence may be genetic, rather than acquired, in origin. An epidemic disease, on the other hand, is a disease that occurs as an 'outbreak', and in the case of prion disease these are the collections of acquired cases like kuru or BSE. Every replicating organism has its 'ecological niche', that is, the place in nature where it survives best, and for the agents of prion disease this frequently involves direct or inadvertent cannibalism. There is, however, another ecological niche in which these agents have found a home. This is the biological laboratory. By transmitting prion disease from natural hosts (sheep and humans) to mice, hamsters, and transgenic mice with modified PrP genes, it has been possible to generate infectious prion proteins with new primary amino acid sequences and new strain characteristics. These new 'strains' are man-made.

'Ice nine'

In his novel *Cat's cradle*, Kurt Vonnegut comments that 'Nothing in this book is true' (Vonnegut 1963). Since the comment is in the book it cannot be true, so there must be something in the book which is true. (This is, of course, Epimenides' paradox. Epimenides, a Cretan, famously said 'All Cretans are liars'.) A major theme of the book is that a tiny seed of a polymer of water has the capacity to change all the water that it encounters into the same polymer. When that water is inside a living creature the effect is, of course, fatal. Once the polymer escaped into the natural world it could not be stopped and the world was destroyed. The idea is based on a phenomenon well known to chemists called 'industrial infection'. Polymers consist of molecules that have stuck together in a crystal structure so that they can form mega-molecules of unlimited size. They are the solid substances such as plastics and synthetic fibres which can be made into cloth. In many cases, however, it is possible to stack the single molecules in a variety of different ways to produce polymers with differing properties. In the case of Kurt Vonnegut's science fiction, the polymer of water (called 'ice-nine') had a melting point of 130° Fahrenheit, which made it incompatible with the existence of life on Earth.

In industrial processes the polymer formed depends partly on the physicochemical conditions prevailing at the time, but in many cases, a 'seed' of one of the forms of the polymer is sufficient to ensure that all the newly synthesized polymer is then of the same form as the seed. There can even be cross-polymerization, where a seed as non-specific as a bit of dust can set off the process of polymerization in a fluid that is ready to polymerize. The industrial production of polymers can be contaminated by unwanted seeds, which lead to changes in the shape of the mega-molecules produced, rendering the plastic product useless. This collapse in the production process can spread from one factory to another if people or goods move between factories, carrying the infectious seeds with them.

One of the problems that evolution has had to solve is to create solid animals from the 'primeval soup' of proteins, carbohydrates, and other chemicals which are essential to life. Hard substances like bone, stretchy substances like ligaments, extremely smooth substances like cartilage, and sticky substances to make cells adhere to each other, are all necessary to produce an animal. (Cancerous cells lose their stickiness so that tumours break up and spread round the body to cause lethal 'secondaries'.) Many proteins make filaments and larger structures by a process called 'self-directed self-assembly', that is, the molecules, once formed, automatically stick together in a particular way, without instructions from elsewhere telling them what to do. It is hardly surprising that the assembly of structures from separate molecules can sometimes go wrong. One of the ways in which things can go wrong results in the production of amyloids. These are very dense, chemically inactive, deposits of polymerized versions of otherwise essential proteins in the body. They cause damage by accumulating, for example in arteries, by failing to do the job of the normal form of the protein, and, sometimes, by being specifically toxic to the cells in which they occur.

There is a variety of chemically different amyloids. The most important to occur in the brain was first described by Alois Alzheimer in 1907 as 'a peculiar substance' in the cerebral cortex in a patient who had died of a severe dementing illness (Alzheimer 1907). This was the first reported case of what is now recognized as the most common cause of dementia in the elderly and is now called either Alzheimer's disease or, to those of a particularly pernickety turn of mind, 'senile dementia of the Alzheimer type'. Although first described at the beginning of the twentieth century, Alzheimer's disease remained a relatively obscure disease until the 1960s, when people began to realize that dementia in old age was a pathological condition that did not occur in everyone, or at least not to the same degree, rather than that dementia was an inevitable product of growing old. The number of people suffering from Alzheimer's disease has increased dramatically as life expectancy has increased. Nancy Reagan did much to stimulate research and debate into this awful illness by freely admitting that ex-President Ronald Reagan was suffering from Alzheimer's disease.

Comparison between Alzheimer's disease and prion disease is worthwhile for many reasons, not least because, in prion disease, PrP is frequently deposited in the brain as an amyloid in a pathological process resembling that seen in Alzheimer's disease (Forloni *et al.* 1996). Both Alzheimer's disease and human prion disease occur in sporadic, familial, and acquired forms. In both diseases, sporadic cases have a mean later age at onset than familial cases, and familial cases are associated with mutations in the genes that make, or are involved in processing, the protein that accumulates as an amyloid. Alzheimer's disease is found in families that carry one of several mutations in the 'amyloid precursor protein' (APP) gene, or in genes that modulate the processing of APP. Familial prion disease is seen in families that carry one of several mutations in the PrP gene. Acquired cases of CJD result from accidental contamination with PrP^{sc}. Acquired Alzheimer's disease (together with other neurological damage) results from head trauma, particularly repeated head trauma, such as that seen in professional boxers.

Metabolic perturbations cause an increase in APP production which results in the production of β-amyloid. The link between prion disease and Alzheimer's disease is brought even closer in the 'Indiana pedigree' of GSS. In affected members of this pedigree the plaques in the brain are composed of PrP-amyloid and the β-amyloid found in Alzheimer's disease. The brains of these patients also contain many neurones bearing 'neurofibrillary tangles'—a deposit of yet another amyloid (tau protein) which is characteristic of Alzheimer's disease. Until the advent of the techniques of immunohistochemistry, the brains of patients from the 'Indiana pedigree' were indistinguishable from those of patients with Alzheimer's disease (Ghetti *et al.* 1989). That prion disease should initiate the deposition of β-amyloid, especially in fairly elderly patients, is perhaps not too surprising since the deposition of β-amyloid in normal ageing, and in response to neurotrauma, suggests that it may be a natural response of the elderly brain to any sort of damage. More shocking has been the recent description of a family with a mutation in the presenilin-1 gene. Mutations within the presenilin-1 gene usually lead to familial Alzheimer's disease, but in the illness associated with this newly reported mutation the plaques were found to contain PrP-amyloid as well as β-amyloid (el-Hachimi *et al.* 1996). It has yet to be demonstrated that transmission can occur using brain tissue from family members.

Prion disease and Alzheimer's disease differ radically in that prion disease is experimentally and accidentally transmissible, whereas Alzheimer's disease is not (although the majority of familial forms of human prion disease, especially those of long duration with the deposition of many PrP-plaques, have not been transmitted experimentally.) The process of corruption of molecules is, none the less, a common theme occurring in both types of disease. In artificial conditions the precursor molecule of β-amyloid, or synthesized portions of that precursor molecule, are biochemically unstable, and may rapidly and unpredictably form β-amyloid fibrils. PrP^{sc} forms PrP-amyloid on extraction from brain, and does so spontaneously within the brain to form amyloid plaques in a proportion (but, importantly, not all) cases of prion disease. Artificially synthesized portions of PrP will also spontaneously polymerize in a test tube. β-Amyloid and PrP^{sc} are both made up structurally of 'β-pleated sheet' formations. Chemical procedures that unfold and refold PrP molecules can be used to manipulate the amount of infectivity associated with an extract of PrP^{sc} (Kocisko *et al.* 1996).

In some cases of familial prion disease it has been possible to show that the protein product of both copies of the PrP gene enter into the disease process (although interestingly in other cases this may not be so). This demonstrates that, just as in acquired cases of prion disease, the normal prion protein can be involved in the disease process, but in this case it is affected by the prion protein produced by the mutated gene. In a disease known as 'hereditary cerebral haemorrhage with amyloidosis, Dutch type', which is caused by a mutation within the APP gene and which is characterized by the accumulation of β-amyloid in the brain, it has also been shown that the β-amyloid is produced from both the abnormal and the normal APP molecules (Gajdusek 1994). This suggests that the β-amyloid, or a pathological pre-amyloid molecule, is recruiting or corrupting normal molecules in a manner that bears some similarities to the crucial pathological process of prion disease. We have found small numbers of β-amyloid plaques in the brains of middle-aged monkeys injected with human brain containing β-amyloid, but not in those injected with other sorts of brain tissue or in age-matched controls (Baker *et al.* 1994).

The most important difference between the pathogenesis of PrP^{sc} and β-amyloid is that infectious PrP^{sc} is probably not, itself, an amyloid (Wille *et al.* 1996). The most rapidly fatal cases of prion disease do not have PrP-amyloid plaques in their brains, and the PrP27–30 which can be extracted from the brain (and which is an amyloid) is made from a non-amyloid form of PrP^{sc} during the extraction process. All amyloidoses require three stages of protein processing. The 'precursor protein', that is the newly synthesized protein, has to be processed by cellular mechanisms which slightly shorten the protein; the shortened form then takes on a β-pleated shape; and these β-pleated molecules then stack together to form fibrils that have the properties of amyloids. APP is known to be processed in at least two different ways, and the relative proportion of each processed product is different in the brains of patients with Alzheimer's disease compared to healthy people. Although mutations in the APP gene alter the probability with which the precursor will be processed by these two pathways, the mechanism of the switch from one pathway to another is not known. In prion disease, PrP^{sc} reacts differently to processing compared to PrP^{c}, so that the processed product of PrP^{sc} may take on a β-pleated shape and, subsequently, accumulate as amyloid deposits in the brain. The events involved in the production of PrP^{sc} and β-amyloid are remarkably similar, but may differ in certain ways that will turn out to be very important when they are understood. We have argued that prion disease is something novel in biology and, in the realm of infection, this is true. It may turn out, however, that the pathogenesis of prion disease is remarkably similar to the pathogenesis of Alzheimer's disease. If this is so, an understanding of prion disease, which kills about 50 people per year in Britain, may enable us to understand Alzheimer's disease, which contributes to the deaths of many thousands.

A cure for prion disease?

The 1980s was the era of 'champagne genetics'. It was commonplace to hear scientists say 'if we can find the gene we will be able to cure the disease'. When, after sometimes years of painstaking work, genes for specific diseases were found, there was great celebration. This was, however, only the beginning of the story rather than the end. Being able to work on the protein that is most involved in producing a disease is extremely useful, but knowing the problem and knowing the answer are not the same thing. From the viewpoint of the more circumspect 1990s, it has to be admitted that the identification of genes linked to diseases has not yet led to any cures for those diseases. Genetic counselling and molecular testing may eliminate inherited disease from a few families, but it is unlikely to eradicate any adult-onset disorder because of the immense personal difficulties of applying the test at a time that is beneficial to the families concerned.

Prion disease was the first neurological disease for which the gene mutations clearly leading to disease were found. The protein in prion disease is well known and well studied, but since the mechanism of the conversion of PrP^c to PrP^{sc} remains as mysterious and elusive as the Holy Grail, there is little prospect at present of halting that process, once it has begun. There may be ways of interfering with the process and slowing it down, but these are not therapeutically attractive since they are likely to keep the patient alive in a seriously debilitated state for a long time. Biochemical methods of interfering with the formation of PrP^{sc} are currently being investigated in tissue cultures as a means of exploring the nature of the interaction between PrP^c and PrP^{sc}. Whether such methods will be of therapeutic value will depend on whether they can be shown to be effective, and not toxic, in infected animals prior to their use in people. Interference with amyloid formation is another current area of interest for the pharmaceutical industry, particularly in developing treatments for Alzheimer's disease. Since the mechanisms of amyloidosis are much the same, irrespective of the particular protein involved, such treatments may inhibit PrP-amyloid formation as well. It is not clear, however, whether in the case of prion disease, this would merely increase the availability of a pre-amyloid infectious protein, and accelerate the disease process. Turning off the PrP gene would undoubtedly prevent or halt prion disease and, since transgenic mice lacking the PrP gene are not grossly abnormal, it might be supposed that turning off the PrP gene would not be deleterious. However, at the present time, there are no ways of turning specific genes on and off at will.

In a wholly other context, Sigmund Freud, commenting on his life's work to a friend, said, 'I often console myself with the idea, that even though we achieve so little therapeutically, at least we understand why more cannot be achieved' (quoted in Shorter 1997). So it is with prion disease. Personal and family tragedies, ethnological catastrophes, and economic disasters can all be traced back to the mischievous misfolding of one small molecule. That this misfolding frequently depends on an error in one of a few letters of the book of the genome is just the way it is.

Glossary of terms

Listed below are some of the terms used in this book. A brief explanation or definition is provided for each. These definitions are not exhaustive and are appropriate to the context of the book.

Aetiology: the cause of a disease. For example, it might be a viral or bacterial infection, or it might result from a genetic defect or an environmental toxin.

Allele: alternative forms of a gene at the same chromosomal location.

Alzheimer's disease: progressive neurodegenerative disease, usually of elderly people. Characteristic neuropathological features in the brain include amyloid plaques (protein deposits) and neurofibrillary tangles.

Amino acids: the building blocks of protein. There are about 20 different amino acids. Proteins may consist of 200–300 amino acids linked together by chemical bonds between one amino acid and the next.

Amyloid: substance (usually protein) deposited in tissues in certain diseases.

Antibody: a protein produced by the body's immune system in response to a foreign or 'non-self' protein. The antibody will combine with the invading protein to inactivate it.

Astrocyte: one of the many types of non-neurone cell found within the nervous system (brain). Astrocytes support the function of neurones.

Astrocytosis: increase in numbers and size of astrocytes as a result of traumatic brain damage or in neurodegenerative disease.

Ataxia: unsteady standing and walking as a result of brain dysfunction.

Atypical prion disease: a form of prion disease in humans.

Autosomal dominant: type of genetic inheritance. An individual carries two copies of each gene on the non-sex chromosomes, and only needs one of these copies to be defective in order to develop disease because the defective gene is dominant over the normal gene.

Autosomal recessive: type of genetic inheritance. The individual needs two copies of the defective gene to develop disease.

Bacterium: single-celled living organisms. Bacteria can reproduce rapidly in the right circumstances and are the cause of a number of diseases, e.g. tuberculosis.

Basal ganglia: a large structure in the middle of the brain concerned with movement.

Bases: the building blocks of nucleic acid. There are five different bases: A, adenine; T, thymine; U, uracil; G, guanine; and C, cytosine. Deoxyribonucleic acid (DNA) contains A, T, G, C; ribonucleic acid contains A, U, G, C. Each base combines with a sugar and a phosphate group to form a nucleotide. Nucleotides combine to form nucleic acid.

Base pair: complementary bases which pair up to form part of the double helical structure of DNA: Adenine pairs with Thymine and Guanine pairs with Cytosine.

Bovine spongiform encephalopathy (BSE): prion disease of cattle.

Cerebellum: brain lobe below and behind the cerebrum: involved in co-ordination and control of movement and balance.

Chimeric: composed (usually) of genetic material from two separate organisms. A chimeric gene may contain sequences from the equivalent gene in two different organisms.

Chromosome: DNA coils found in all the cells of the body. Chromosomes contain all the genes. Each cell carries two copies of each chromosome except the sex cells (ovum and sperm), which carry one copy. There are 22 pairs of non-sex chromosomes (autosomes), one X chromosome and one Y chromosome. An ovum has 22 autosomes and an X chromosome: a sperm has 22 autosomes and an X or a Y chromosome. When a sperm fertilizes an ovum the resulting cell will have the full complement of 22 pairs of autosomes and either 2 X chromosomes (female offspring) or one X and one Y chromosome (male offspring).

Chronic wasting disease (CWD): prion disease of mule deer and Rocky Moutain elk.

Codon: sequence of three bases in the DNA which specifies a particular amino acid during protein synthesis.

Contagious: transfer of disease from one individual to another by physical contact.

Cortex: the cerebral cortex is the outer layer of the brain, containing neurones. It is involved in early processing of incoming information such as vision, hearing, etc., as well as motor output.

Creutzfeldt–Jakob disease (CJD): prion disease of humans.

Dementia: loss of higher mental faculties such as learning, reasoning, and remembering.

Deoxyribonucleic acid (DNA): the informational molecule in every cell: specifies the sequence of amino acids in every protein during protein synthesis.

Donor: in the context of this book, the animal or human with prion disease used as a source of infectious agent in transmission experiments.

Dura mater: part of the membrane covering the brain (cf. Meninges).

Electroencephalogram (EEG): a graphic display of brain electrical activity. The EEG pattern is usually abnormal in CJD.

Endemic: endemic diseases occur continuously within a population.

Enzyme: proteins that catalyse specific chemical reactions within a cell. There are many thousands of different enzymes.

Epidemic: epidemic diseases occur as outbreaks within the population.

Familial: occurring within families.

Fatal familial insomnia (FFI): a prion disease of humans.

Foré: one of the many language groups spoken in Papua New Guinea. The kuru epidemic affected mainly the Foré-speaking people.

Gene: the unit of heredity consisting of a DNA sequence. Each gene specifies the amino acid sequence of a particular protein.

Genetic: relating to gene. A genetic disease results from a defect in a gene.

Genome: the entire genetic material of the cell.

Genotype: the genetic information within a cell; takes account of genetic variations. Used to describe different forms of a specific gene (more correctly allelotype).

Gerstmann–Sträussler–Scheinker disease (GSS): prion disease of humans.

Gliosis: proliferation of non-neuronal glial cells in the brain in response to brain damage.

Growth hormone: a chemical produced in the pituitary gland and essential for normal growth.

Heterodimer: a complex of two dissimilar proteins.

Heterozygote: carrying two different alleles at the same location on a pair of chromosomes.

Homogenize: to blend tissue in a small version of a household culinary blender.

Homozygote: carrying identical alleles at the same location on two different alleles.

Host: the recipient of infectious material in transmission experiments.

Huntington's disease: a fatal, autosomal dominant genetic disease in humans. Characterized, clinically, by involuntary movements with progressive dementia, and, neuropathologically, by loss of tissue in part of the brain called the basal ganglia.

Iatrogenic: literally, caused by the doctor. Iatrogenic disease is cause by medical mishap.

Idiopathic: description of a disease arising, literally, 'from within'. A disease without obvious external cause or known genetic basis.

Immune response: the body's ability to recognize foreign proteins, especially those associated with viruses and bacteria, and to attack those proteins, thereby fighting off infections.

Immunohistochemistry: technique for identifying proteins in sections of tissues. Makes use of antibodies to specific proteins. When the antibody attaches to the protein of interest, a chemical coupled to the antibody allows the distribution of the antibody, and therefore the protein, to be visualized.

Incubation period: in the context of this book, the time between infection of the host and clinical signs of disease.

Infectious: transfer of disease from one individual to another by a number of routes, including airborne.

Intraneuronal vacuolation: small holes within neurones, seen with a high-power microscope; found only in spongiform encephalopathy.

Kuru: prion disease of humans in Papua New Guinea.

Lesion profile: in the context of this book, the distribution of pathological changes within the brain of an animal with prion disease.

Meat-and-bone meal: dried material rich in protein, produced by rendering animal carcasses. Used as animal feed supplement until banned in the UK. Also used as fertilizer.

Meninges: the outer membrane covering the brain.

Molecule: the smallest particle of a particular substance. In the context of this book, the smallest unit of a protein.

Mutation: a change in the DNA sequence of a gene, usually as a result of faulty copying during cell division. If a mutation occurs in the sex cells (germline) it will be inherited. Some mutations lead to disease.

Myoclonus: involuntary brief contraction of the muscles, leading to a limb jerk.

Neurodegeneration: progressive damage to the nerve cells (neurones) leading to cell death.

Neurofibrillary tangle: a deposit of insoluble proteins within nerve cells (neurones). Characteristic feature of Alzheimer's disease.

Neurone: nerve cell. Specialized cell in the brain which usually transmits information to other cells.

Nucleotide: see Base.

Obligate carrier: an individual who must be carrying a specific gene mutation. Usually someone who is no longer available to be tested for the mutation but in whom mutation is inferred because of their position within the family.

Parkinson's disease: a neurodegenerative disease in the elderly, characterized by tremor and an inability to initiate movements.

Pathogen: an agent that causes disease, e.g. a virus or a toxin.

Pathogenesis: the evolution of a disease. The processes underlying the course of disease.

Pathogenic: causing disease.

Peptide: the term usually refers to a small number of amino acids linked together. A peptide with a large number of amino acids is a polypeptide.

Phenotype: the appearance of an organism resulting from an interaction between the genes and the environment.

Pituitary gland: a small structure in the base of the brain which produces hormones.

Plaque: characteristic appearance of protein deposit (amyloid) in brain. Plaques are seen in Alzheimer's disease and some cases of prion disease, although the protein deposited is different in each disease.

Polymorphism: non-pathogenic variations in a gene (alleles) which are common in the population. The prion protein gene is polymorphic in humans.

Post-translational modification: an alteration in the structure of a protein after it has been synthesized.

Primary sequence: the sequence of amino acids in a protein determined by the sequence of codons in the gene for that protein.

Prion protein: the protein at the centre of the prion diseases. In the healthy animal or human it can be digested by a protease enzyme. In animals or humans with prion disease, prion protein has been post-translationally modified so that it is now resistant to protease digestion. Now known as PrP. See also PrP^c and PrP^{sc}.

Prions: a name given to molecules of the abnormal form of prion protein. According to the prion hypothesis, prions are the pathogens in prion diseases.

Protease K: one of a group of enzymes, the proteases, which can digest (cut) proteins down to their constituent amino acids.

Protein: a major class of large biological molecules. Proteins are composed of hundreds of amino acids. They may consist of a single polypeptide (see above) or a number of polypeptides bound together. They act as enzymes catalysing reactions in the cell or as part of the structure of the cell. The primary structure of the protein is the sequence of amino acids in the protein. Sections of the polypeptide chain fold to take up different shapes (e.g. a helical twist or a flat sheet) referred to as the secondary structure. The whole protein then folds up on itself to yield the 'finished' molecule. This is the tertiary structure.

Proteinaceous: composed of protein.

PrP: general term for the product of the prion protein gene. Can exist in normal or abnormal form.

PrP^c: normal form of prion protein found in many tissues, especially in brain. Associated with neurones. Its function is unknown.

PrP gene: the gene that codes for prion protein. In humans it is located on chromosome 20 and in mice it is on chromosome 2.

PrP^{sc}: abnormal form of prion protein found in brains of animals and humans with prion disease.

Rendering: the process by which animal remains are boiled, dried, and converted into a protein-rich powder for inclusion in animal feedstuff.

Replication: process by which viruses make identical copies of themselves.

Restriction enzyme: type of enzyme widely used in molecular biology. Restriction enzymes cut nucleic acids at very specific sites determined by the sequence of bases.

Scrapie: the prion disease of sheep.

Scrapie-associated fibrils (SAFs): small clumps of twisted fibres seen (using the electron microscope) in extracts of brain from animals and humans with prion disease. Main constituent is abnormal prion protein. Originally identified in scrapie-affected brain.

Secondary structure: proteins consist of a string of amino acids which take on a secondary structure of helices, loops, and ribbons.

Specified bovine offals: bovine tissues excluded from food in the UK by law. Includes brain, spinal cord, intestines, spleen, thymus, and a number of other organs.

Spongiform change: extraneuronal vacuolation typical of, but not definitively diagnostic of, prion disease.

Spongiform encephalopathy (SE): term reserved for the neuropathology of prion diseases. Comprises spongiform change, intraneuronal vacuolation, neuronal cell loss, and astrocytosis. In some cases of prion disease, the degree of SE may be minimal.

Sporadic: occurring without an identifiable precipitating event.

Strain of agent: term used to explain why different preparations of SE agent cause different lesion profiles and incubation periods in various strains of mice.

Strain of mouse: genetically different types of mice.

Tangle: see Neurofibrillary tangle.

Tertiary structure: the final three-dimensional shape of a protein.

Thalamus: large mass of grey matter in the brain which receives information from sensory inputs and relays it to sensory cortical areas.

Transcription: the process whereby information is transmitted from chromosomal DNA to messenger RNA.

Transgene: a gene from an animal of one species which is inserted into the genome of an animal of another species.

Transgenic: carrying transgenes, as in transgenic mice which carry human PrP genes.

Translation: process whereby the information in messenger RNA is converted into protein structure.

Transmissible: able to cause disease if it gains access to another host. If brain tissue from a human with spongiform encephalopathy is injected into the brain of an animal, the animal will develop spongiform encephalopathy.

Transmissible mink encephalopathy (TME): epidemic spongiform encephalopathy of ranch-bred mink. There have been a number of such outbreaks, thought to be caused by feeding scrapie-infected sheep or sheep products to the mink.

Vacuole: a small, clear region in tissue seen under the microscope. In spongiform encephalopathy, there are intraneuronal vacuoles visible with a high-power microscope, together with extraneuronal vacuoles visible with a low-power microscope.

Virino: hypothetical infectious agent. Suggested by scientists working with mouse-adapted scrapie to account for apparent mutations in the scrapie agent and the existence of a number of different agent strains.

Virus: small infectious agent consisting of an informational molecule (RNA or DNA) encased within a protein coat. Having infected a cell, the virus has all the information necessary to make identical copies of itself, although it needs to use the cell's mechanisms for synthesis.

Wild type: the common form of a gene found in the general population.

References

Adam, J., Crow, T. J., Duchen, L. W., Scaravilli, F., and Spokes, E. (1982). Familial cerebral amyloidosis and spongiform encephalopathy. *Journal of Neurology, Neurosurgery and Psychiatry*, **45**, 37–45.

Adams, D. (1979). *The hitch hiker's guide to the galaxy.* Pan Books, London.

Alpers, M. P. (1968). Kuru: implications of its transmissibility for the interpretation of its changing epidemiological pattern. In *The central nervous system, some experimental models of neurological diseases,* (ed. O. T. Baile and D. E. Smith), pp. 234–51. Williams and Wilkins, Baltimore.

Alpers, M. (1992). Reflections and highlights: a life with kuru. In *Prion diseases of humans and animals,* (ed. S. B. Prusiner, J. Collinge, J. Powell, and B. Anderton), pp. 66–76. Ellis Horwood, Chichester.

Alzheimer, A. (1907). Über eine eigenartige Erkrankung der Hirnrinde. *Centralblatt fur Nervenheilkunde und Psychiatrie*, **30**, 177–9.

Anderson, R. M., Donnelly, C. A., Ferguson, N. M., Woolhouse, M. E. J., Watt, C. J., Udy, H. J. *et al.* (1996). Transmission dynamics and epidemiology of BSE in British cattle. *Nature*, **382**, 779–88.

Arens, W. (1979). *The man-eating myth; anthropology and anthropophagy.* Oxford University Press, New York.

Baker, H. F. and Ridley, R. M. (ed.) (1996). *Prion diseases.* Humana Press, New Jersey.

Baker, H. F., Ridley, R. M., and Crow, T. J. (1985). Experimental transmission of an autosomal dominant spongiform encephalopathy: does the infectious agent originate in the human genome? *British Medical Journal*, **291**, 299–302.

Baker, H. F., Ridley, R. M., and Wells, G. A. H. (1993). Experimental transmission of BSE and scrapie to the common marmoset. *Veterinary Record*, **132**, 403–6.

Baker, H. F., Ridley, R. M., Duchen, L. W., Crow, T. J., and Bruton, C. J. (1994). Induction of β-amyloid in primates by injection of Alzheimer's disease brain homogenate: comparison with transmission of spongiform encephalopathy. *Molecular Neurobiology*, **8**, 25–40.

Baker, H. F., Ridley, R. M., Wells, G. A. H., and Ironside, J. W. (1996). Spontaneous spongiform encephalopathy in a monkey. *Lancet*, **348**, 955–6.

Bateman, D., Hilton, D., Loce, S., Zeidler, M., Beck, J., and Collinge, J. (1995). Sporadic Creutzfeldt–Jakob disease in an 18-year-old in the UK. *Lancet*, **346**, 1155–6.

Beck, E., Daniel, P. M., and Parry, H. B. (1964). Degeneration of the cerebellar and hypothalamo-neurohypophyseal systems in sheep with scrapie and its relationship to human system degenerations. *Brain*, **87**, 153–76.

Beck, E., Daniel, P. M., Gajdusek, D. C., and Gibbs, C. J. (1969). Similarities and differences in the pattern of pathological changes in scrapie, kuru, experimental kuru and subacute polioencephalopathy. In *Virus diseases of the nervous system*, (ed. C. W. M. Whitty, J. T. Hughes, and F. O. MacCallum), pp. 107–20. Blackwell Scientific Press, Oxford.

Bell, J. E. (1996). Neuropathological diagnosis of human prion disease; PrP immunocytochemical techniques. In *Prion diseases*, (ed. H. F. Baker and R. M. Ridley), pp. 59–83. Humana Press, New Jersey.

Bell, J. E. and Ironside, J. W. (1993). How to tackle a possible Creutzfeldt–Jakob disease necropsy. *Journal of Clinical Pathology*, **46**, 193–7.

Bessen, R. A., Kocisko, D. A., Raymond, G. J., Nandan, S., Lansbury, P. T., and Caughey, B. (1995). Non-genetic propagation of strain-specific properties of scrapie prion protein. *Nature*, **375**, 698–700.

Bons, N., Mestre-Francés, N., Charnay, Y., and Tagliavini, F. (1996). Spontaneous spongiform encephalopathy in a young rhesus monkey. *Lancet*, **348**, 55.

Brandner, S., Isenmann, S., Raeber, A., Fischer, M., Sailer, A., Kobayashi, Y. *et al.* (1996*a*). Normal host prion protein necessary for scrapie-induced neurotoxicity. *Nature*, **379**, 339–43.

Brandner, S., Raeber, A., Sailer, A., Blättler, T., Fischer, M., Weissmann, C. *et al.* (1996*b*). Normal host prion protein (PrP^c) is required for scrapie spread within the central nervous system. *Proceedings of the National Academy of Sciences USA*, **93**, 13148–51.

Britton, T. C., Al-Sarraj, S., Shaw, C., Campbell, T. and Collinge, J. (1995). Sporadic Creutzfeldt–Jakob disease in a sixteen-year-old in the UK. *Lancet*, **346**, 1155.

Brown, P. (1988). Human growth hormone therapy and Creutzfeldt–Jakob disease: a drama in three acts. *Pediatrics*, **81**, 85–92.

Brown, P. (1996). Environmental causes of human spongiform encephalopathy. In *Prion diseases,* (ed. H. F. Baker and R. M. Ridley), pp. 139–54. Humana Press, New Jersey.

Brown, P. and Cathala, F. (1979). Creutzfeldt–Jakob disease in France. In *Slow transmissible diseases of the nervous system*, Vol. 1, (ed. S. B. Prusiner and W. J. Hadlow), pp. 213–27. Academic Press, New York.

Brown, P., Cervenáková, L., Boellaard, J. W., Stavrou, D., Goldfarb, L. G., and Gajdusek, D. C. (1994). Identification of a PRNP gene mutation in Jakob's original Creutzfeldt–Jakob disease family. *Lancet*, **344**, 130–1.

Bruce, M. E., Chree, A., McConnell, I., Foster, J., Pearson, G., and Fraser, H. (1994). Transmission of bovine spongiform encephalopathy and scrapie to mice: strain variation and the species boundary. *Philosophical Transactions of the Royal Society, London B, Biological Sciences*, **343**, 405–11.

Bruce, M. E., Will, R. G., Ironside, J. W., McConnell, I., Drummond, D., Suttie, A., *et al.* (1997). Transmissions to mice indicate that 'new variant' CJD is caused by the BSE agent. *Nature*, **389**, 498–501.

Büeler, H., Aguzzi, A., Sailer, A., Greiner, R.-A., Autenreid, P., Aguet, M. *et al.* (1993). Mice devoid of PrP are resistant to scrapie. *Cell,* **73**, 1339–47.

Butler, D. (1996). Did UK 'dump' contaminated feed after ban. *Nature,* **381**, 544–5.

Cameron, E. and Crawford, A. D. (1974). A familial neurological disease complex in a Bedfordshire community. *Journal of the Royal College of General Practitioners,* **24**, 435–6.

Caughey, B., Kocisko, D. A., Priola, S. A., Raymond, G. J., Race, R. E., Bessen, R. A. *et al.* (1996). Methods for studying prion protein (PrP) metabolism and the formation of protease-resistant PrP in cell culture and cell-free systems. In *Prion diseases,* (ed. H. F. Baker and R. M. Ridley), pp. 285–99. Humana Press, New Jersey.

Chandler, R. L. (1961). Encephalopathy in mice produced by inoculation with scrapie brain material. *Lancet,* **i**, 1378–9.

Chazot, G., Brousolle, E., Lapras, C., Blättler, T., Aguzzi, A., and Kopp, N. (1996). New variant of Creutzfeldt–Jakob disease in a 26-year-old French man. *Lancet,* **347**, 1181.

Collinge, J., Palmer, M. S., and Dryden, A. J. (1991). Genetic predisposition to iatrogenic Creutzfeldt–Jakob disease. *Lancet,* **337**, 1441–2.

Collinge, J., Brown, J., Hardy, J., Mullan, M., Rossor, M. N., Baker, H. F. *et al.* (1992). Inherited prion disease with 144 base pair gene insertion. 2. clinical and pathological Features. *Brain,* **115**, 687–710.

Collinge, J., Palmer, M. S., Sidle, K. C. L., Hill, A. F., Gowland, I., Meads, J. *et al.* (1995). Unaltered susceptibility to BSE in transgenic mice expressing human prion protein. *Nature,* **378**, 779–83.

Collinge, J., Sidle, K. C. L., Meads, J., Ironside, J. W., and Hill, A. F. (1996). Molecular analysis of prion protein strain variation and the aetiology of 'new variant' CJD. *Nature,* **383**, 685–90.

Connolly, J. H., Allen, I. V., and Dermott, E. (1988). Transmissible agent in the amyotrophic form of Creutzfeldt–Jakob disease. *Lancet,* **ii**, 1459–60.

Creutzfeldt, H. G. (1920). Über eine eigenartige herdförmige Erkrankung des Zentralnervensystems. *Zeitschrift für die gestamte Neurologie und Psychiatrie,* **57**, 1–18.

Cuillé, J. and Chelle, P. L. (1936). La maladie dite tremblante du mouton est-elle inoculable? *Comptes Rendus de Academie des Sciences (Paris),* **203**, 1552–4.

Davies, P. T. G., Jahfar, S., and Ferguson, I. T. (1993). Creutzfeldt–Jakob disease in individual occupationally exposed to BSE. *Lancet,* **342**, 680.

Dawkins, R. (1976). *The selfish gene.* Oxford University Press, Oxford.

Delasnerie-Laupretre, N., Poser, S., Pocchiari, M., Wientjens, D. P. W. M., and Will, R. G. (1995). Creutzfeldt–Jakob disease in Europe. *Lancet,* **346**, 898.

Denny, G. O. and Hueston, W. D. (1997). Epidemiology of bovine spongiform encephalopathy in Northern Ireland 1988–1995. *Veterinary Record,* **140**, 302–6.

Derkatch, I. L., Chernoff, Y. O., Kushnirov, V. V., Inger-Vechtonov, S. G., and

Liebman, S. W. (1996). Genesis and variability of [PSI] prion factors in *Saccharomyces cerevisiae*. *Genetics*, **144**, 1375–86.

Dickinson, A. G. and Outram, G. W. (1979) The scrapie replication-site hypothesis and its implications for pathogenesis In *Slow transmissible diseases of the nervous system*, Vol. 2, (ed. S. B. Prusiner and W. L. Hadlow), pp. 13–31. Academic Press, New York.

Dickinson, A. G., Young, G. B., Stamp, J. T., and Renwick, C. C. (1965). An analysis of natural scrapie in Suffolk sheep. *Heredity*, **20**, 485–503.

Diringer, H., Beekes, M., and Oberdieck, U. (1994). The nature of the scrapie agent: the virus theory. *Annals of the New York Academy of Science*, **724**, 246–58.

Forloni, G., Tagliavini, F., Bugiano, O., and Salmona, M. (1996). Amyloid in Alzheimer's disease and prion-related encephalopathies: studies with synthetic peptides. *Progress in Neurobiology*, **49**, 287–315.

Foster, J. D., McKelvey, W. A., Mylne, M. J., Williams, A., Hunter, N., Hope, J. *et al.* (1992). Studies on maternal transmission of scrapie in sheep by embryo transfer. *The Veterinary Record*, **130**, 341–3.

Foster, J. D., Hunter, N., Williams, A., Mylne, M. J. A., McKelvey, W. A. C., Hope, J. *et al.* (1996). Observations on the transmission of scrapie in experiments using embryo transfer. *The Veterinary Record*, **138**, 559–62.

Fraser, H., McBride, P. A., Scott, J. R., Hunter, N., and Foster, J. D. (1989). Scrapie, models and homologues. *State Veterinary Journal*, **43**, 11–22.

Gajdusek, D. C. (1990). Subacute spongiform encephalopathies: transmissible cerebral amyloidosis caused by unconventional viruses. In *Virology*, (2nd edn), (ed. B. N. Fields, D. M. Knipe, R.M. Chanock, M.S. Hirsch, J. L. Melnick, T. P. Monath *et al.*), pp. 2289–324. Raven Press, New York.

Gajdusek, D. C. (1994). Nucleation of amyloidogenesis in infectious amyloidoses of brain. *Annals of the New York Academy of Science*, **724**, 173–90.

Gajdusek, D. C., Gibbs, C. J., and Alpers, M. P. (1966). Experimental transmission of a kuru-like syndrome to chimpanzees. *Nature*, **209**, 794–6.

Gerstmann, J., Sträussler, E., and Scheinker, I. (1936). Über eine eingenartige hereditär-familiäre Erkrankung des Zentralnervensystems. Zugleich ein Beitag zur Frage des vorzeitigen lokalen Alterns. *Zeitschrift für Neurologie*, **154**, 736–62.

Ghetti, B., Tagliavini, F., Masters, C. L., Beyreuther, K., Giaconne, G., Verga, L. *et al.* (1989). Gerstmann–Sträussler–Scheinker disease. II. Neurofibrillary tangles and plaques with PrP-amyloid coexist in an affected family. *Neurology*, **39**, 1453–61.

Ghetti, B., Tagliavini, F., Hsiao, K., Dlouhy, S. R., Yee, R. D., Giaccone, G. *et al.* (1992). Indiana variant of Gerstmann–Sträussler–Scheinker disease. In *Prion diseases of humans and animals*, (ed. S. B. Prusiner, J. Collinge, J. Powell, and B. Anderson), pp. 154–67. Ellis Horwood, Chichester, UK.

Gibbs, C. J. (1992). Spongiform encephalopathies—slow, latent, and temporate virus infections—in retrospect. In *Prion diseases of humans and animals*, (ed. S. B. Prusiner, J. Collinge, J. Powell, and B. Anderton), pp. 53–62. Ellis Horwood, Chichester.

Gibbs, C. J., Gajdusek, D. C., Asher, D. M., Alpers, M. P., Beck, E., Daniel, P. M., and Matthews, W. B. (1968). Creutzfeldt–Jakob disease (spongiform encephalopathy): transmission to the chimpanzee. *Science*, **161**, 388–9.

Glasse, R. M. (1967). Cannibalism in the kuru region of New Guinea. *Transactions of the New York Academy of Sciences*, **29**, 748–54.

Goldberg, H., Alter, M., and Kahana, E. (1979). The Libyan Jewish focus of Creutzfeldt–Jakob disease: a search for the mode of natural transmission. In *Slow transmissible diseases of the central nervous system,* Vol. 1, (ed. S. B. Prusiner and W. J. Hadlow), pp. 195–211. Academic Press, New York.

Goldfarb, L. G., Petersen, R. B., Tabaton, M., Brown, P., LeBlanc, A. C., Montagna, P. *et al.* (1992). Fatal familial insomnia and familial Creutzfeldt–Jakob disease: disease phenotype determined by a DNA polymorphism. *Science*, **258**, 806–8.

Gray, J. R., Soldan, J. R., and Harper, P. S. (1996). Special problems of genetic counselling in adult-onset diseases. In *Prion diseases,* (ed. H. F. Baker and R. M. Ridley), pp. 199–210. Humana Press, New Jersey.

Griffiths, J. S. (1967). Self-replication and scrapie. *Nature*, **215**, 1043–4.

el Hachimi, K. H., Cervenáková, L., Brown, P. Goldfarb, L. G., Rubenstein, R., Gajdusek, D. C. *et al.* (1996). Mixed features of Alzheimer's disease and Creutzfeldt–Jakob disease in a family with a presenilin-1 mutation on chromosome 14. *International Journal of Clinical Investigation*, **3**, 223–33.

Hadlow, W. J. (1959). Scrapie and kuru. *Lancet*, **2**, 289–90.

Hadlow, W. J. (1991). To a better understanding of natural scrapie. In *Sub-acute spongiform encephalopathies,* (ed. R. Bradley, M. Savey, and B. Marchant), pp. 117–30. Kluwer Academic Publishers, Dordrecht, The Netherlands.

Hadlow, W. J., Race, R. E., and Kennedy, R. C. (1979). Natural infection of sheep with scrapie virus. In *Slow transmissible diseases of the nervous system*, Vol. 2, (ed. S. B. Prusiner and W. J. Hadlow), pp. 3–12. Academic Press, New York.

Hadlow, W. J., Kennedy, R. C., and Race, R. E. (1982). Natural infection of Suffolk sheep with scrapie virus. *Journal of Infectious Diseases*, **146**, 657–64.

Hainfellner, J. A., Liberski, P. P., Guiroy, D. C., Cervenáková, L., Brown, P., Gajdusek., D. C. *et al.* (1997). Pathology and immunocytochemistry of a kuru brain. *Brain Pathology*, **7**, 547–53.

Harries-Jones, R., Knight, R., Will, R. G., Coussens, S., Smith, P. G., and Matthews, W. B. (1988). CJD in England and Wales, 1980–1984: a case-control study of potential risk factors. *Journal of Neurology, Neurosurgery and Psychiatry*, **51**, 1113–19.

Herzberg, L., Herzberg, R. N., Gibbs, C. J., Sullivan, W., Amyx, H., and Gajdusek, D. C. (1974). Creutzfeldt–Jakob disease: hypothesis for high incidence in Libyan Jews in Israel. *Science*, **186**, 848.

Hill, A. F., Desbruslais, M., Joiner, S., Sidle, K. C. L., Gowland, I., Collinge, J., *et al.* (1997). The same prion strain causes vCJD and BSE. *Nature*, **389**, 448–50.

Hornabrook, R. W. (1979). Kuru and clinical neurology. In *Slow transmissible diseases of the nervous system,* Vol. 1, (ed. S. B. Prusiner and W. J. Hadlow), pp. 37–66. Academic Press. New York.

Hornabrook, R. W. and Wagner, F. (1975). Creutzfeldt–Jakob disease. *Papua New Guinea Medical Journal,* **18**, 226–8.

Hourrigan, J. L. (1990). Experimentally induced bovine spongiform encephalopathy in cattle in Mission, Texas, and the control of scrapie. *Journal of the American Veterinary Medical Association,* **196**, 1678–9.

Hourrigan, J. L., Klingsporn, A., Clark, W. W., and de Camp, M. (1979). Epidemiology of scrapie in the United States. In *Slow transmissible diseases of the nervous system,* Vol. 1, (ed. S. B. Prusiner and W. J. Hadlow), pp. 331–56. Academic Press, New York.

Howard, R. S. (1996). Creutzfeldt–Jakob disease in a young woman. *Lancet,* **347**, 945–8.

Hsiao, K., Baker, H. F., Crow, T. J., Poulter, M., Owen, F., Terwilliger, J. D. *et al.* (1989). Linkage of a prion protein missense variant to Gerstmann–Sträussler syndrome. *Nature,* **337**, 342–5.

Hsiao, K. K., Scott, M., Foster, D., Groth, D. F., DeArmond, S. J., and Prusiner, S. B. (1990). Spontaneous neurodegeneration in transgenic mice with mutant prion protein of Gerstmann–Sträussler syndrome. *Science,* **250**, 1587–90.

Hsiao, K. K., Groth, D., Scott, M., Yang, S.-L., Serban, H., Rapp, D. *et al.* (1994). Serial transmission in rodents of neurodegeneration from transgenic mice expressing mutant prion protein. *Proceedings of the National Academy of Sciences USA,* **91**, 9126–30.

Hunter, N., Foster, J. D., Goldmann, W., Stear, M. J., Hope, J., and Bostock, C. (1996). Natural scrapie in a closed flock of Cheviot sheep occurs only in specific PrP genotypes. *Archives of Virology,* 141, 809–24.

Hunter, N., Cairns, D., Foster, J. D., Smith, G., Goldmann, W., and Donelly, K. (1997). Is scrapie a solely genetic disease? *Nature,* **386**, 137.

Ironside, J. W. (1996*a*). Neuropathological diagnosis of human prion disease; morphological studies. In *Prion diseases,* (ed. H. F. Baker and R. M. Ridley), pp. 35–57. Humana Press, New Jersey.

Ironside, J. W. (1996*b*). Human prion diseases. *Journal of Neural Transmission (Suppl),* **47**, 231–46.

Jakob, A. (1921). Über eine der multiplen Sklerose klinisch nahestehende Erkrankung des Zentralnervensystems (spastische Pseudosklerose) mit bemerkenwertem anatomischem Befunde. Mitteilung eines vierten Falles. *Medizinische Klinik,* **17**, 372–6.

Kirkwood, J. K., Cunningham, A. A., Wells, G. A. H., Wilesmith, J. W., and Barnett, J. E. F. (1993). Spongiform encephalopathy in a herd of greater kudu (*Tragelaphus strepsiceros*): epidemiological observations. *Veterinary Record,* **133**, 360–4.

Kirschbaum, W. R. (1968). *Jakob–Creutzfeldt disease.* Elsevier, New York.

Klitzman, R. L., Alpers, M. P., and Gajdusek, D. C. (1984). The natural incubation period of kuru and the episodes of transmission in three clusters of patients. *Neuroepidemiology*, **3**, 3–20.

Kocisko, D. A., Lansbury, P. T., and Caughey, B. (1996). Partial unfolding and refolding of scrapie-associated prion protein: evidence for a critical 16-kDa C-terminal domain. *Biochemistry*, **35**, 13434–42.

Kolata, G. (1986). Anthropologists suggest cannibalism is a myth. *Science*, **232**, 1497–500.

Kretzchmar, H. A., Honold, G., Seitelberger, F., Feucht, M., Wessely, P., Mehraein, P. *et al.* (1991). Prion protein mutation in family first reported by Gerstmann, Sträussler and Scheinker. *Lancet*, **337**, 1160.

Kuhn, T. S. (1962). *The structure of scientific revolutions*. University of Chicago Press, London.

Lacey, R. W. (1994). *Mad cow disease: a history of BSE in Britain*. Cypsela Publications, St Helier, Jersey, CI.

Lancet (1996). Betraying the public over nvCJD risk. *Lancet*, **348**, 1529.

Lasmézas, C. I., Deslys, J. P., Demainay, P., Adjou, K. T., Lamoury F., Dormont, D. *et al.* (1996). BSE transmission to macaques. *Nature*, **383**, 743–4.

Lehmann, S. and Harris, D. A. (1996). Two mutant prion proteins expressed in cultured cells acquire biochemical properties reminiscent of the scrapie isoform. *Proceedings of the National Academy of Sciences USA*, **93**, 5610–14.

Liberski, P. P. (1990). Ultrastructural neuropathological features of bovine spongiform encephalopathy. *Journal of the American Veterinary and Medical Association*, **196**, 1682.

McArthur, J. R. (1953). Patrol report. Department of Native Affairs, Port Moresby, Papua New Guinea.

MacDonald, S. T., Sutherland, K., and Ironside, J. W. (1996). Prion protein genotype and pathological phenotype studies in sporadic Creutzfeldt–Jakob disease. *Neuropathology and Applied Neurobiology*, **22**, 285–92.

Manson, J. L., Clarke, A. R., McBride, P. A., McConnell, I., and Hope, J. (1994). PrP dosage determines the timing but not the final intensity or distribution of lesions in scrapie pathology. *Neurodegeneration*, **3**, 331–40.

Marsh, R. F. (1992). Transmissible mink encephalopathy. In *Prion diseases of animals and humans*, (ed. S. B. Prusiner, J. Collinge, J. Powell, and B. Anderton), pp. 300–7. Ellis Horwood, Chichester.

Masters, C. L. and Richardson, E. P. (1978). Subacute spongiform encephalopathy (Creutzfeldt–Jakob disease). The nature and progression of spongiform change. *Brain*, **101**, 333–4.

Masters, C. L., Harris, J. O., Gajdusek, D. C., Gibbs, C. J., Bernoulli, C., and Asher, D. M. (1979). Creutzfeldt–Jakob disease: patterens of worldwide occurrence and the significance of familial and sporadic clustering. *Annals of Neurology*, **5**, 177–88.

Masters, C. L, Gajdusek, D. C., and Gibbs, C. J. (1981*a*). The familial occurrence of Creutzfeldt–Jakob disease and Alzheimer's disease. *Brain*, **104**, 535–58.

Masters, C. L., Gajdusek, D. C., and Gibbs, C. J. (1981b). Creutzfeldt–Jakob disease virus isolations from the Gerstmann–Sträussler syndrome with an analysis of the various forms of amyloid plaque deposition in the virus-induced spongiform encephalopathies. *Brain*, **104**, 559–88.

Matthews, W. B. (1985). Creutzfeldt–Jakob disease. *British Medical Journal*, **291**, 483.

Medawar, P. S. (1957). *The uniqueness of the individual*. Methuen, London.

Merz, P. A., Somerville, R. A., Wisniewski, H. M., and Iqbal, K. (1981) Abnormal fibrils from scrapie-infected brain. *Acta Neuropathologica*, **54**, 63–74.

Meyer, A., Leigh, D., and Bagg, C. E. (1954). A rare presenile dementia associated with cortical blindness (Heidenhain's syndrome). *Journal of Neurology, Neurosurgery and Psychiatry*, **17**, 129–33.

Moore, R. C., Redhead, N. J., Selfridge, J., Hope, J., Manson, J. C., and Melton, D. W. (1995). Double replacement gene targetting for the production of a series of mouse strains with different prion protein gene alterations. *Biotechnology*, **13**, 999–1004.

Morgan, K. L., Nicholas, K., Glover, M. J., and Hall, A. P. (1990). A questionnaire survey of the prevalence of scrapie in sheep in Britain. *Veterinary Record*, **127**, 373–6.

Narang, H. (1996). Origin and implications of bovine spongiform encephalopathy. *Proceedings of the Society for Experimental Biology and Medicine*, **211**, 306–22.

Nevin, S., McMenemey, W. H., Behrman, S., and Jones, D. P. (1960). Subacute spongiform encephalopathy—a subacute form of encephalopathy attributable to vascular dysfunction (spongiform cerebral atrophy). *Brain*, **83**, 519–69.

Oesch, B., Westaway, D., Wälchli, M., McKinley, M. P., Kent, S. B. H., Aebersold, R. *et al.* (1985). A cellular gene encodes scrapie PrP 27–30 protein. *Cell*, **40**, 735–46.

Owen, F., Poulter, M., Lofthouse, R., Collinge, J., Crow T. J., Risby, D. *et al.* (1989). Insertion in the prion protein gene in familial Creutzfeldt–Jakob disease. *Lancet*, **i**, 51–2.

Palmer, A. C. (1959). Scrapie, a review of the literature. *Veterinary Reviews and Annotations*, **5**, 1–15.

Palmer, A. C. (1960). Scrapie, a nervous disease of sheep characterised by pruritus. In *Progress in the biological sciences in relation to dermatology*, (ed. A. Rook), pp. 239–43. Cambridge University Press, Cambridge.

Palmer, M. S., Dryden, A. J., Hughes, J. T., and Collinge, J. (1991). Homozygous prion protein genotype predisposes to sporadic Creutzfeldt–Jakob disease. *Nature*, **352**, 340–2.

Parchi, P., Capellari, S., Chen, S. G., Petersen, R. B., Gambetti, P., Kopp, N. *et al.* (1997). Typing prion isoforms. *Nature*, **386**, 232–3.

Parry, H. B. (1962). Scrapie: a transmissible and hereditary disease of sheep. *Heredity*, **17**, 75–105.

Parry, H. B. (1983). *Scrapie disease in sheep*. Academic Press, London.

Pattison, I. H. (1974). Scrapie in sheep selectively bred for high susceptibility. *Nature*, **248**, 594–5.

Pattison, I. H. (1988). Fifty years with scrapie: a personal reminiscence. *Veterinary Record*, **123**, 661–6.

Pattison, I. H. (1992). A sideways look at scrapie: 1732–1991. In *Prion diseases of humans and animals*, (ed. S. B. Prusiner, J. Collinge, J. Powell, and B. Anderton), pp. 15–22. Ellis Horwood, Chichester.

Pattison, I. H. and Jones, K. M. (1967). The possible nature of the transmissible agent of scrapie. *Veterinary Record*, **80**, 1–8 .

Popper, K. R. (1959). *The logic of scientific discovery*. Hutchinson, London. (Reprinted by Routledge 1992.)

Poulter, M., Baker, H. F., Frith, C. D., Leach, M., Lofthouse, R., Ridley, R. M. *et al.* (1992). Inherited prion disease with 144 base pair gene insertion. 1. Genealogical and molecular studies. *Brain*, **115**, 675–85.

Prusiner, S. B. (1982). Novel proteinaceous infectious particles cause scrapie. *Science*, **216**, 136–44.

Prusiner, S. B. (1992). Prion biology. In *Prion diseases of humans and animals*, (ed. S. B. Prusiner, J. Collinge, J. Powell, and B. Anderton), pp. 533–67. Ellis Horwood, Chichester.

Prusiner, S. B. (1994). Biology and genetics of prion diseases. *Annual Reviews in Microbiology*, **48**, 655–86.

Prusiner, S. B. (ed). (1996). Prions, prions, prions. *Current Topics in Microbiology and Immunology*, **207**, 1–160.

Prusiner, S. B. (1997). Cell biology and transgenic models of prion diseases. In *Prion diseases,* (ed. J. Collinge and M. S. Palmer), pp. 130–62. Oxford University Press, Oxford.

Prusiner, S. B., Scott, M., Foster, D., Pan, K. M., Groth, D., Mirenda, C. *et al.* (1990). Transgenetic studies implicate interactions between homologous PrP isoforms in scrapie prion replication. *Cell*, **63**, 673–86.

Ridley, R. M. and Baker, H. F. (1995). The myth of maternal transmission of spongiform encephalopathy. *British Medical Journal*, **311**, 1071–5.

Ridley, R. M. and Baker, H. F. (1996*a*). No maternal transmission? *Nature*, 384, 17.

Ridley, R. M. and Baker, H. F. (1996*b*). To what extent is strain variation evidence for an independent genome in the agent of the transmissble spongiform encephalopathies? *Neurodegeneration*, **5**, 219–31.

Ridley, R. M. and Baker, H. F. (1997). The nature of transmission in prion diseases. *Neuropathology and Applied Neurobiology*, **23**, 273–80.

Ridley, R. M., Baker, H. F., and Crow, T. J. (1986). Transmissible and non-transmissible neurodegenerative disease; similarities in age of onset and genetics in relation to aetiology. *Psychological Medicine*, **16**, 199–207.

Rosenthal, N. P., Keesey, J., Crandall, B., and Brown, J. (1976). Familial neurological disease associated with spongiform encephalopathy. *Archives of Neurology*, **33**, 252–9.

Sawcer, S. J., Yuill, G. M., Esmonde, T. F. G., Ironside, J. W., and Bell, J. E. (1993). Creutzfeldt–Jakob disease in an individual occupationally exposed to BSE. *Lancet*, **341**, 642.

Scull, A. T. (1982). *Museums of madness.* Penguin Books, London.

Shorter, E. (1997). *A history of psychiatry.* John Wiley and Sons, New York.

Sigurdarson, S. (1991). Epidemiology of scrapie in Iceland and experience with control measures. In *Sub-Acute spongiform encephalopathies*, (ed. R. Bradley, M. Savey, and B. Marchant), pp. 233–42. Kluwer Academic Publisher, Dordrecht, The Netherlands.

Smith, P. E. M., Zeidler, M., Ironside, J. W., Estibeiro, P., and Moss, T. H. (1995). Creutzfeldt–Jakob disease in a dairy farmer. *Lancet*, **346**, 898.

Steele, T. W. (1964). *The control and possible eradication of natural scrapie. IV. The practical problems of flockmasters.* Report of a Scrapie Seminar, United States Department of Agriculture, ARS, Washington, DC.

Stockman, S. (1913). Scrapie: an obscure disease of sheep. *Journal of Comparative Pathology and Therapeutics*, **26**, 317–27.

Taylor, D. M., Dickinson, A. G., Fraser, H., Robertson, P. A., Salacinski, P. R., and Lowry, P. J. (1985). Preparation of growth hormone free from contamination with unconventional slow viruses. *Lancet*, **ii**, 260–2.

Telling, G. C., Haga, T., Torchia, M., Tremblay, P., DeArmond, S. J., and Prusiner, S. B. (1996a). Interactions between wild-type and mutant prion proteins modulate neurodegeneraion in transgenic mice. *Genes and Development*, **10**, 1736–50.

Telling, G. C., Parchi, P., DeArmond, S. J., Cortelli, P., Montagna, P., Gabizon, R. *et al.* (1996b). Evidence for the conformation of the pathologic isoform of the prion protein encyphering and propagating prion diversity. *Science*, **274**, 2079–82.

Vonnegut, K. (1963). *Cat's cradle.* Penguin, London.

Wells, G. A. H. and Wilesmith, J. W. (1995). The neuropathology and epidemiology of bovine spongiform encephalopathy. *Brain Pathology*, **5**, 91–103.

Wells, G. A. H., Scott, A. C., Johnson, C. T., Gunning, R. F., Hancock, R. D., Jeffrey, M. *et al.* (1987). A novel progressive spongiform encephalopathy in cattle. *Veterinary Record*, **121**, 419–20.

Westaway, D., Neuman, S., Zuliani, V., Mirenda, C., Foster., Detwiler, L. *et al.* (1992). Transgenic approaches to experimental and natural prion diseases. In *Prion diseases of humans and animals*, (ed. S. B. Prusiner, J. Collinge, J. Powell, and B. Anderton), pp. 473–82. Ellis Horwood, Chichester.

Westaway, D., Zuliani, V., Cooper, C. M., Da Costa, M., Neuman, S., Jenny, A. L. *et al.* (1994a). Homozygosity for prion protein alleles encoding glutamine-171 renders sheep susceptible to natural scrapie. *Genes and Development*, **8**, 959–69.

Westaway, D., DeArmond, S. J., Cayetano, C. J., Groth, C. J., Foster, D., Yang, S. L. *et al.* (1994b). Degeneration of skeletal muscle, peripheral nerves, and the central nervous system in transgenic mice overexpressing wild-type prion proteins. *Cell*, **76**, 117–29.

Wilesmith, J. W., Wells, G. A. H., Cranwell, M. P., and Ryan, J. B. M. (1988). Bovine spongiform encephalopathy: epidemiological studies. *Veterinary Record*, **123**, 638–44.

Will, R. G. (1987). Transmissible dementia: epidemiology. In *Degenerative neurological disease in the elderly,* (ed. R. A. Griffiths and S. T. McCarthy), pp. 101–18. John Wright, Bristol.

Will, R. G. and Matthews, W. B. (1981). Creutzfeldt–Jakob disease in a lifelong vegetarian. *Lancet*, **ii**, 937.

Will, R. G. and Matthews, W. B. (1984). A retrospective study of Creutzfeldt–Jakob disease in England and Wales 1970–1979 I: clinical features. *Journal of Neurology, Neurosurgery and Psychiatry*, **47**, 134–40.

Will, R. G., Matthews, W. B., Smith, P. G., and Hudson, C. (1986). A retrospective study of Creutzfeldt–Jakob disease in England and Wales II: epidemiology. *Journal of Neurology, Neurosurgery and Psychiatry*, **49**, 749–55.

Will, R. G., Ironside, J. W., Zeidler, M., Cousens, S. N., Estibeiro, K., Alperovitch, A. et al. (1996). A new variant of Creutzfeldt–Jakob disease in the UK. *Lancet*, **347**, 921–5.

Wille, H., Zhang, G. F., Baldwin, M. A., Cohen, F. E., and Prusiner, S. B. (1996). Separation of scrapie prion infectivity from PrP amyloid polymers. *Journal of Molecular Biology*, **259**, 608–21.

Williams, E. S. and Young, S. (1980). Chronic wasting disease of captive mule deer: a spongiform encephalopathy. *Journal of Wildlife Diseases*, **16**, 89–98.

Williams, E. S. and Young, S. (1982). Spongifrom encephalopathy of Rocky Mountain elk. *Journal of Wildlife Diseases*, **18**, 465–71.

Worster-Drought, C., Greenfield, J. G., and McMenemy, W. H. (1944). A form of familial presenile dementia with spastic paralysis. *Brain*, **67**, 38–43.

Wyatt, J. M., Pearson, G. R., Smerdon, T. N., Gruffydd-Jones, T. J., Wells, G. A. H., and Wilesmith, J. W. (1991). Naturally occurring scrapie-like spongiform encephalopathy in five domestic cats. *Veterinary Record*, **129**, 233–6.

Zigas, V. (1990). *Laughing death; the untold story of kuru.* Humana Press, New Jersey.

Recommended reading

Books

Baker, H. F. and Ridley, R. M. (ed.) (1996). *Prion diseases.* Humana Press, New Jersey.

Collinge, J. and Palmer, M. S. (ed.) (1997). *Prion diseases.* Oxford University Press, Oxford.

Kimberlin, R. H. (ed.) (1976). *Slow virus diseases of animals and man.* North Holland, Amsterdam.

Lacey, R. W. (1994). *Mad cow disease: a history of BSE in Britain.* Cypsela Publications, St Helier, Jersey.

Parry, H. B. (1983). *Scrapie disease in sheep.* Academic Press, London.

Prusiner, S. B. and Hadlow, W. J. (ed.) (1979). *Slow transmissible diseases of the nervous system*, Vols 1 and 2. Academic Press, New York.

Prusiner, S. B. and McKinley, M. P. (ed.) (1987). *Prions. Novel infectious pathogens causing scrapie and Creutzfeldt–Jakob disease.* Academic Press, San Diego.

Prusiner, S. B., Collinge, J., Powell, J., and Anderton, B. (ed.) (1992). *Prion diseases of humans and animals.* Ellis Horwood, Chichester.

General reviews

Prusiner, S. B. (1992). Prion biology. In *Prion diseases of animals and humans,* (ed. S. B. Prusiner, J. Collinge, J. Powell, and B. Anderton), pp. 533–67. Ellis Horwood, Chichester.

Prusiner, S. B. (1994). Biology and genetics of prion diseases. *Annual Reviews in Microbiology*, **48**, 655–86.

Prusiner, S. B. (1996). Molecular biology and pathogenesis of prion diseases. *Trends in Biochemical Sciences*, **21**, 482–7.

Schreuder, B. E. C. (1993). General aspects of transmissible spongiform encephalopathies and hypotheses about the agents. *Veterinary Quarterly*, **15**, 167–74.

Schreuder, B. E. C. (1994). Animal spongiform encephalopathies—an update. Part I. Scrapie and lesser known animal spongiform encephalopathies. *Veterinary Quarterly*, **16**, 174–81.

Schreuder, B. E. C. (1994). Animal spongiform encephalopathies—an update. Part II. Bovine spongiform encephalopathy (BSE). *Veterinary Quarterly*, **16**, 182–92.

Other views

Carp, R. I., Meeker, H., and Sersen, E. (1997). Scrapie strains retain their distinctive characteristics following passages of homogenates from different brain regions and spleen. *Journal of General Virology*, **78**, 283–90.

Diringer, H., Beekes, M., and Oberdieck, U. (1994). The nature of the scrapie agent. *Annals of the New York Academy of Sciences*, **724**, 246–58.

Kimberlin, R. H. (1996). Speculations on the origin of BSE and the epidemiology of CJD. In *Bovine spongiform encephalopathy*, (ed. C. J. Gibbs), pp. 155–75. Serono Symposia USA, Norwell, Mass.

Lacey, R. W. and Dealler, S. F. The transmission of prion disease. *Human Reproduction*, **9**, 92–1800.

Narang. H. (1996). The nature of the scrapie agent: the virus theory. *Proceedings of the Society for Experimental Biology and Medicine*, **212**, 208–24.

Özel, M., Xi, Y. G., Baldauf, E., Diringer, H., and Pocchiari, M. (1994). Small virus-like structure in brains from cases of sporadic and familial Creutzfeldt–Jakob disease. *Lancet*, **344**, 923–4.

Purdey, M. (1996). The UK epidemic of BSE: slow virus or chronic pesticide-initiated modification of the prion protein? *Medical Hypotheses*, **46**, 429–54.

Scrapie

Clark, A. M., Moar, J. A. E., and Nicholson, J. T. (1994). Diagnosis of scrapie. *Veterinary Record*, **130**, 377–8.

Foster, J. D. and Dickinson, A. G. (1988). The unusual properties of CH1641, a sheep-passaged isolate of scrapie. *Veterinary Record*, **123**, 5–8.

Hadlow, W. J. (1995). Neuropathology and the scrapie-kuru connection. *Brain Pathology*, **5**, 27–31.

Hunter, N., Moore, L., Hosie, B. D., Dingwall, W. S., and Greig, A. (1997). Association between natural scrapie and PrP genotype in a flock of Suffolk sheep in Scotland. *Veterinary Record*, **140**, 59–63.

Parsonson, I. M. (1996). Scrapie: recent trends. *Australian Veterinary Journal*, **74**, 2–6.

Westaway, D., Zuliani, V., Cooper, C. M., Da Costa, M., Neumann, S., Jenny, A. L. *et al.* (1994). Homozygosity for prion protein alleles encoding glutamine-171 renders sheep susceptible to natural scrapie. *Genes and Development*, **8**, 959–69.

Prion disease in animals other than sheep and cows

Goldman, W., Martin, T., Foster, J., Hughes, S., Smith, G., Hughes, K. *et al.* (1996). Novel polymorphisms in the caprine PrP gene: a codon 142 mutation associated with scrapie incubation period. *Journal of General Virology*, **77**, 2885–91.

Kirkwood, J. K. and Cunningham, A. A. (1994). Epidemiological observations on spongiform encephalopathies in captive wild animals in the British Isles. *Veterinary Record*, **135**, 296–303.

Lowenstein, D. H., Butler, D. A., Westaway, D., McKinley, M. P., DeArmond, S. J., and Prusiner, S. B. (1990). Three hamster species with different scrapie incubation times and neuropathological features encode distinct prion proteins. *Molecular and Cellular Biology*, **10**, 1153–63.

Marsh, R. F., Bessen, R. A., Lehmann, S., and Hartshough, G. R. (1991). Epidemiological and experimental studies on a new incident of transmissible mink encephalopathy. *Journal of General Virology*, **72**, 589–94.

Williams, E. S. and Young, S. (1993). Neuropathology of chronic wasting disease of mule deer (*Odocoileus hemionus*) and elk (*Cervus elaphus nelsoni*). *Veterinary Pathology*, **30**, 36–45.

Wood, J. L. N., Done, S. H., Pritchard, C. G., and Wooldridge, M. J. A. (1992). Natural scrapie in goats; case histories and clinical signs. *Veterinary Record*, **131**, 66–8.

BSE

Foster, J. D., Hope, J., and Fraser, H. (1993). Transmission of bovine spongiform encephalopathy to sheep and goats. *Veterinary Record*, **133**, 339–41.

Hoinville, L. J., Wilesmith, J. W., and Richards, M. S. (1995). An investigation of risk factors for cases of bovine spongiform encephalopathy born after the introduction of the 'feed ban'. *Veterinary Record*, **136**, 312–18.

Wells, G. A. H. and Wilesmith, J. W. (1995). The neuropathology and epidemiology of bovine spongiform encephalopathy. *Brain Pathology*, **5**, 91–103.

Wells, G. A. H., Wilesmith, J. W., and McGill, I. A. (1991). Bovine spongiform encephalopathy: a neuropathological perspective. *Brain Pathology*, **1**, 69–78.

Wilesmith, J. W. and Ryan, J. B. M. (1992). Bovine spongiform encephalopathy: epidemiological studies on the origin. *Veterinary Record*, **128**, 199–203.

Kuru

Alpers, M. P. (1992). Kuru. In *Human biology in Papua New Guinea: the small cosmos*, (ed. R. D. Attenborough and M. P. Alpers), pp. 313–34. Oxford University Press, Oxford.

Prusiner, S. B., Gajdusek, D. C., and Alpers, M. P. (1982). Kuru with incubation periods exceeding two decades. *Annals of Neurology*, **12**, 1–9.

Scrimgeour, E. M., Masters, C. L., Alpers, M. P., Kaven, J., and Gajdusek, D. C. (1983). A clinicopathological study of a case of kuru. *Journal of Neurological Sciences*, **59**, 265–75.

Iatrogenic Creutzfeldt–Jakob disease

Bernoulli, C., Siegfried, J., Baumgartner, G., Regli, F., Rabinowicz, T., Gajdusek, D. C. *et al.* (1977). Danger of accidental person-to-person transmission of Creutzfeldt–Jakob disease by surgery. *Lancet*, **i**, 478–9.

Brown, P. (1996). Environmental causes of human spongiform encephalopathy. In *Prion diseases*, (ed. H. F. Baker and R. M. Ridley), pp. 139–54. Humana Press, New Jersey.

Brown, P., Cervenáková, L., Goldfarb, L. G., McCombie, W. R., Rubenstein, R., Will, R. G. *et al.* (1994). Iatrogenic Creutzfeldt–Jakob disease: an example of the interplay between ancient genes and modern medicine. *Neurology*, **44**, 291–3.

Duffy, P., Wolf, J., Collins, G., DeVoe, A. G., Streeten, B., and Cowen, D. (1974). Possible person-to-person transmission of Creutzfeldt–Jakob disease. *New England Journal of Medicine*, **290**, 692–3.

Esmonde, T., Lueck, C. J., Symon, L., Duchen, L. W., and Will, R. G. (1993). Creutzfeldt–Jakob disease and lyophilised dura mater grafts: report of two cases. *Journal of Neurology, Neurosurgery and Psychiatry*, **56**, 999–1000.

Markus, H. S., Duchen, L. W., Parkin, E. M., Kurtz, A. B., Jacobs, H. S., Costa, D. C. *et al.* (1992). Creutzfeldt–Jakob disease in recipients of human growth hormone in the United Kingdom: a clinical and radiographic study. *Quarterly Journal of Medicine*, **82**, 43–51.

Nevin, S., McMenemy, W. H., Behrman, S., and Jones, D. P. (1960). Subacute spongiform encephalopathy—a subacute form of encephalopathy attributable to vascular dysfunction (spongiform cerebral atrophy). *Brain*, **83**, 519–64.

Will, R. G. and Matthews, W. B. (1982). Evidence for case-to-case transmission of Creutzfeldt–Jakob disease. *Journal of Neurology, Neurosurgery and Psychiatry*, **45**, 235–8.

Creutzfeldt–Jakob disease

Brown, P., Cathala, F., Castaigne, P., and Gajdusek, D. C. (1986). Creutzfeldt–Jakob disease: clinical analysis of a consecutive series of 230 neurpathologically verified cases. *Annals of Neurology*, **20**, 597–602.

Brown, P., Rodgers-Johnson, P., Cathala, F., Gibbs, C. J., and Gajdusek, D. C. (1984). Creutzfeldt–Jakob disease of long duration: clinicopathological characteristics, transmissibility, and differential diagnosis. *Annals of Neurology*, **16**, 295–304.

Brown, P., Gibbs, C. J., Rodgers-Johnson, P., Asher, D. M., Sulima, M. P., Bacotre, A. *et al.* (1994). Human spongiform encephalopathy: the National Institutes of Health series of 300 cases of experimentally transmitted disease. *Annals of Neurology*, **35**, 513–29.

Genetics of human prion disease

Brown, P., Goldfarb, L. G., Kovanen, J., Haltia, M., Cathala, F., Sulima, M. P. *et al.* (1992). Phenotypic characteristics of familial Creutzfeldt–Jakob disease associated with the codon-178 Asn PRNP mutation. *Annals of Neurology*, **31**, 282–5.

Collinge, J., Poulter, M., Davis, M. B., Baraitser, M., Owen, F., Crow, T. J. *et al.* (1991). Presymptomatic detection or exclusion of prion protein gene defects in families with inherited prion diseases. *American Journal of Human Genetics*, **49**, 1351–4.

Dlouhy, S. R., Hsiao, K., Farlow, M. R., Foroud, T., Conneally, P. M., Johnson, P. *et al.* (1992). Linkage of the Indiana kindred of Gerstmann–Sträussler–Scheinker disease to the prion protein gene. *Nature Genetics*, **1**, 64–7.

Goldfarb, L. G., Korczyn, A. D., Brown, P., Chapman, J., and Gajdusek, D. C. (1990). Mutation in codon 200 of the scrapie amyloid precursor gene linked to Creutzfeldt–Jakob disease in Sephardic Jews of Libyan and non-Libyan origin. *Lancet*, **336**, 637–8.

Goldfarb, L. G., Brown, P., McCombie, W. R., Goldgaber, D., Swergold, G. D., Wills, P. R. *et al.* (1991). Transmissible familial Creutzfeldt–Jakob disease associated with five, seven, and eight extra octapeptide coding repeats in the PRNP gene. *Proceedings of the National Academy of Sciences USA*, **88**, 10926–30.

Hsiao, K. K., Cass, C., Schellenberg, G. D., Bird, T., Gage D. E., Wisniewski, H. *et al.* (1991). A prion protein variant in a family with the telencephalic form of Gerstmann–Sträussler–Scheinker syndrome. *Neurology*, **41**, 681–4.

Kitamoto, T., Iizuka, R., and Tateishi, J. (1993). An amber mutation of prion protein in Gerstmann–Sträussler syndrome with mutant PrP plaques. *Biochemical Biophysical Research Communications*, **191**, 709–14.

Prion protein biochemistry

Barry, R. A. and Prusiner, S. B. (1986). Monoclonal antibodies to the cellular and scrapie prion proteins. *Journal of Infectious Diseases*, **154**, 518–21.

Basler K., Oesch, B., Scott, M., Westaway, D., Wälchli., M., Groth, D. F. *et al.* (1986). Scrapie and cellular PrP isoforms are encoded by the same chromosomal gene. *Cell*, **46**, 417–28.

Borchelt, D. R., Scott, M., Taraboulos, A., Stahl, N., and Prusiner, S. B. (1990). Scrapie and cellular prion proteins differ in their kinetics of synthesis and topology in cultured cells. *Journal of Cellular Biology*, **110**, 743–52.

Chesebro, B., Race, R., Wehrly, K., Nishio, J., Bloom, M., Lechner, D. *et al.* (1985). Identification of scrapie prion protein-specific mRNA in scrapie-infected and uninfected brain. *Nature*, **315**, 331–33.

Prusiner, S. B., Groth, D. F., Bolton, D. C., Kent, S. B., and Hood, L. E. (1984). Purification and structural studies of a major scrapie prion protein. *Cell*, **38**, 127–34.

Sparkes, R. S., Simon, M., Cohn, V.H., Fournier, R. E. K., Lem, J., Klisak, I. *et al.* (1986). Assignment of the human and mouse prion protein genes to homologous chromosomes. *Proceedings of the National Academy of Sciences USA*, **83**, 7358–62.

Prion protein amyloid

Bockman, J. M., Kingsbury, D. T., McKinley M. P., Bendheim, P. E., and Prusiner, S. B. *et al.* (1985). Creutzfeldt–Jakob disease prion proteins in human brains. *New England Journal of Medicine*, **312**, 73–8.

DeArmond, S. J., McKinley, M. P., Barry, R. A., Braunfeld, M. B., McColloch, J. R., and Prusiner, S. B. (1985). Identification of prion amyloid filaments in scrapie-infected brain. *Cell*, **41**, 221–35.

Gabizon, R., McKinley, M. P., Groth, D. F., Kenaga, L., and Prusiner, S. B. (1987). Purified prion proteins and scrapie infectivity copartition into liposomes. *Proceedings of the National Academy of Sciences USA*, **84**, 4017–21.

Kitamoto, T., Tateishi, J., Tashima, I., Takeshita, I., Barry, R. A., DeArmond, S. J. *et al.* (1986). Amyloid plaques in Creutzfeldt–Jakob disease stain with prion protein antibodies. *Annals of Neurology*, **20**, 204–8.

Prusiner, S. B., McKinley, M. P., Bowman, K. A., Bolton, D. C., Bendheim, P. E., Groth, D. F. *et al.* (1983). Scrapie prions aggregate to form amyloid-like rods. *Cell*, **35**, 349–58.

Wille, H., Baldwin, M. A., Cohen, F. E., DeArmond, S. J., and Prusiner, S. B. (1996). Prion protein amyloid: separation of scrapie infectivity from PrP polymers. In *The nature and origin of amyloid fibrils,* (ed. G. R. Bock and J. A. Goode), pp. 181–99. John Wiley and Sons, Chichester, UK.

Transgenic animals

Scott, M., Foster, D., Mirenda, C., Serban, D., Coufal, F., Wälchli, M., *et al.* (1989). Transgenic mice expressing hamster prion protein produce species-specific scrapie infectivity and amyloid plaques. *Cell*, **59**, 84–857.

Scott, M., Groth, D., Foster, D., Torchia, M., Yang, S.-L., DeArmond, S. J. *et al.* (1993). Propagation of prions with artificial properties in transgenic mice expressing chimeric PrP genes. *Cell*, **73**, 979–88.

Telling, G., Scott, M., Hsiao, K., Foster, D., Yang, S.-L., Torchia, M. *et al.* (1994). Transmission of Creutzfeldt–Jakob disease from human to transgenic mice expressing chimaeric human–mouse prion protein. *Proceedings of the National Academy of Sciences USA*, **91**, 9936–40.

Telling, G., Scott, M., Mastrianni, J., Gabizon, R., Torchia, M., Sidle, K. C. L. *et al.* (1995). Prion propagation in mice expressing human and chimaeric PrP transgenes implicates the interaction of cellular PrP with another protein. *Cell*, **83**, 79–90.

Westaway, D., Mirenda, C. A., Foster, D., Zebarjadian, Y., Scott, M., Torchia, M. *et al.* (1991). Paradoxical shortening of scrapie incubation times by expression of prion protein transgenes derived from long incubation period mice. *Neuron*, **7**, 59–68.

Prion protein folding

Forloni, G., Tagliavini, F., Bugiano, O., and Salmona, M. (1996). Amyloid in Alzheimer's disease and prion-related encephalopathies: studies with synthetic peptides. *Progress in Neurobiology*, **49**, 287–315.

Gassett, M., Baldwin, M. A., Fletterick, R. J., and Prusiner, S. B. (1993). Perturbation of the secondary structure of the scrapie prion protein under conditions associated with changes in infectivity. *Proceedings of the National Academy of Sciences USA*, **90**, 1–5.

Huang, Z., Gabriel, J.-M., Baldwin, M. A., Fletterick, R. J., Prusiner, S. B., and Cohen., F. E. (1994). Proposed three-dimensional structure for the cellular prion protein. *Proceedings of the National Academy of Sciences USA*, **91**, 7139–43.

Kocisko, D. A., Lansbury, P. T., and Caughey, B. (1996). Partial unfolding and refolding of scrapie-associated prion protein: evidence for a critical 16-kDa C-terminal domain. *Biochemistry*, **35**, 13434–42.

Pan, K. M., Baldwin, M., Nguyen, J., Gassett, M., Serban, A., Groth, D. *et al.* (1993). Conversion of α-helices into β-sheets features in the formation of the scrapie prion proteins. *Proceedings of the National Academy of Sciences USA*, **90**, 10962–6.

Safar, J., Roller, P., Gajdusek, D. C., and Gibbs, C. J. (1994). Scrapie amyloid (prion) protein has the conformational characteristics of an aggregated molten globule folding intermediate. *Biochemistry*, **33**, 8375–83.

Tatzelt, J., Prusiner, S. B., and Wech, W. J. (1996). Chemical chaperones interfere with the formation of scrapie prion protein. *EMBO Journal*, **15**, 6363–73.

Index

α-helices 113
Adam, Jane 77
agent strain 144–7
agent strain typing 193
Aguzzi, Adriano 141
Alpers, Michael 42, 55, 101
Alzheimer, Alois 216
Alzheimer's disease 216–17
amyloid 14, 52, 84–6, 110, 217–18
APD, *see* prion disease, atypical
Australia 33

β-amyloid, *see* amyloid
β-pleated sheet 113, 217
β-protein, *see* amyloid
BABs 166–7
Beck, Elisabeth 55, 65
Bell, Jeanne 91, 93
born after the ban, *see* BABs
bovine spongiform encephalopathy, *see* BSE
brainstem 23
Brown, Paul 61, 71
Bruce, Moira 145
BSE 7, 149
    cause 155, 198–9
    Channel Islands 155
    epidemiology 7, 151–4, 166, 199
    experimental transmission 82, 161–2,
        164, 186
    Europe 171–3
    maternal transmission 174–7, 203–4
    public attitudes 8–9, 177–8
    risk to man 163–4, 196–7, 204–6
    secrecy 202–3
    eradication 173–4, 200

cats 168
Caughey, Byron 143
cell-free conversion 143–4
Chandler, Dick 98
chimpanzees 54, 163
CJD 66
    amyotrophic 87
    Brownell–Oppenheimer variant 67
    case P.S. 76–7
    cause 69–71

diagnostic criteria 73, 92
farmers 94
Heidenhain variant 67, 122
iatrogenic 6, 58–64
Nevin–Jones variant 67
new variant, *see* nvCJD
surveillance 89–91
Surveillance Unit 91–4, 179, 189
teenagers 94
Collinge, John 130, 193–4
corneal grafting 58
counselling, genetic 119–21
Creutzfeldt, Hans 66
Creutzfeldt–Jakob disease, *see* CJD

Dawkins, Richard 208–9
Dealler, Stephen 156
Dickinson, Alan 31, 101, 105
Diringer, Heino 103
Duchen, Leo 82
dura mater 64

eland 169
embryo transfer 34–5
export ban 172
extended common source epidemic 153

fatal familial insomnia, *see* FFI
feline spongiform encephalopathy, *see* cats
FFI 2, 68, 87, 96, 131, 146–7
florid plaques, *see* plaques
FSE, *see* cats
Fraser, Hugh 145, 153
Freud, Sigmund 220

Gajdusek, Carleton 42, 55, 79
gemsbok 154, 169
gene 114–15
    blackmail 213
    Faustian 213
    senescence 212
genetic testing 118–22
Gerstmann–Sträussler–Scheinker disease, *see*
    GSS
Gibbs, Joe 54–5

Glasse, Robert 5, 42
Glasse, Shirley 42
goats 26–7
Gordon, W.S. 20
GSS 2, 83–7, 96, 127
    'W' family 77–82, 117–19
    case J.C. 78, 84
    case J.W. 79
    Indiana pedigree 86–7, 128

Hadlow, Bill 30, 53
heterodimer 137
heterozygote advantage 213–14
Hornabrook, Richard 50–1
Hourrigan, Jim 25
Hsiao, Karen 117
human gonadotrophin 64
human growth hormone 60–4
Hunter, Nora 176
hypothalamus 23

Ironside, James 91, 93

Jakob, Alfons 66

Kirschbaum, Walter 67
Klatzo, Igor 65
Kocisko, David 143
kudu 168–70
kuru 4
    and cannibalism 44–7, 57
    and feasts 47–50
    disappearance 56–8
    medicalization 52
    origin 43–4
    sorcery 44
    transmission 54–5

Lacey, Richard 156
Lansbury, Peter 143
Libyan Jews 74–6
Lofhouse, Ray 123–5
louping ill 20

Manson, Jean 139–40
marmosets, see BSE, experimental transmission
Marsh, Richard 35
Masters, Colin 71–3, 83
Matthews, Brian 74, 89–90

meal, meat-and-bone 154
mechanically recovered meat 192
Medawar, Sir Peter 210
Merz, Pat 14, 105
mink 35
mule deer 35
mutation, see PrP gene

neuronal vacuolation 23
neurosurgery 59
New Guinea, see Papua New Guinea
New Zealand 33–4
nucleic acid, 114
nvCJD 170, 179–80
    age at onset 181–2
    and BSE 85, 190–4
    clinical symptoms 182–3
    in France 187
nyala 154, 169

Okapa 42, 52
oryx 169
ostrich 188

Palmer, Tony 38, 188
Papua New Guinea 4, 40–2
paradigm shift 11–12
Parry, James 18, 31, 55, 100
Pattison, Iain 27, 70
pituitary glands 60, 62–3
placentas 28
plaques 84, 132, 184–7
polymerization 84, 215–16
Poulter, Mark 123–5
prion disease 13, 214, 217
    acquired 1, 9–10
    atypical 2, 68, 96, 125
    cure 219–20
    familial 1, 9–10, 117–18
    historical 126
    sporadic 1, 9–10
    today 96–7
prion gene, see PrP gene
prion hypothesis 113, 137–41
prion protein 13, 135
prions 12, 134, 207
PrP gene 15, 107–8, 115, 129–30, 211
    codon 102 mutation 117–18, 127
    codon 178 mutation 131
    codon 198 mutation 128

codon 129 polymorphism 129–31, 147, 196, 214
  insertion mutation 122, 127–8
Prp 27–30: 106–7, 193–4, 217–18
PrP^c 13–16, 108, 112
PrP^{sc} 13–16, 108, 112, 193–4, 217–18
PrP^{sc} typing 193–4
Prusiner, Stan 12, 82, 106, 117, 134

rendering 154, 155–7, 198
Rocky Mountain elk 36
Ruminant Feed Ban 158–9, 199–201

SAF, see scrapie-associated fibrils
SBO Ban 30, 160, 165, 199–210
scrapie 7, 213
  clinical signs 22
  experimental transmission 20, 37
  field cases 21
  genetic susceptibility 32–4
  history 17–20
  lateral transmission 25
  maternal transmission 27, 30–2, 175–6
  neuropathology 22–3
scrapie-associated fibrils 14, 105
SEAC 160, 170
sheep
  Cheviot 33–4, 213
  Herdwick 33
  Suffolk 33–4, 213
  Swaledale 33
Southwood Committee 158–9, 205

Southwood, Sir Richard 158
species barrier 162
Specified Bovine Offals Ban, see SBO Ban
Spongiform Encephalopathy Advisory
    Committee, see SEAC
Stamp, John 101
status spongiosus 23

tangles 85
30 Month Scheme 171
tissue culture 142–3
TME 35–6
transgenic mice 138–41, 147–8, 192–3
transmissible mink encephalopathy, see TME
transplants 141–2
Tyrrell Committee 159–60, 203

virino 104–5
virus 99, 101–3, 208
  slow 70
  thin veneer 80
  unconventional 70
Vonnegut, Kurt 215

Weissmann, Charles 139, 141
Wells, Gerald 150, 161, 164
Westaway, David 33, 138
Wilesmith, John 151
Will, Bob 89, 159

Zigas, Vincent 4, 42